Concise Medical Textbooks

## Respiratory Medicine

# Concise Medical Textbooks

# Respiratory Medicine

## David C. Flenley

BSc, PhD, MB, FRCP(Ed), FRCP

*Professor of Respiratory Medicine,*
*University of Edinburgh*

Baillière Tindall · London

A Baillière Tindall book published by
Cassell Ltd,
35 Red Lion Square, London WC1R 4SG

and at Sydney, Auckland, Toronto, Johannesburg

an affiliate of
Macmillan Publishing Co. Inc.
New York

First published 1981

ISBN 0 7020 0840 0


Filmset in Monophoto Plantin
by Mid-County Press, London SW15
Printed in Great Britain by Mansell (Bookbinders) Ltd, Witham, Essex

**British Library Cataloguing in Publication Data**
Flenley, David C.
  Respiratory medicine. — (Concise medical
  textbooks)
  1. Respiratory organs — Diseases
  I. Title    II. Series

  ISBN 0-7020-0840-0

# Contents

# Preface

If the aim of medicine is the healing of the sick, the clinician, who is the 'combat zone operative' in this process, must try to be jack of many trades; but must be master of one, the art of diagnosis and management. This small book aims to provide the basic knowledge for this demanding endeavour in one of the commonest fields of human disease. Clearly, the remorseless increase in the length of the art is not matched by the life time available to acquire it, so that in a short book some dogmatism is inevitable. This book aims to synthesize the causes and pathogenesis of respiratory disease with the clinical presentations, diagnostic features and management. The text is intended for both senior medical students and candidates for higher qualifications in medicine. It is also hoped that the book will interest general physicians who inevitably are concerned with most of the patients who present with disease of the respiratory system. Experts in this field, and those in need of authoritative reference works, are now well served, notably by *Respiratory Diseases* by John Crofton and Andrew Douglas (1981, 3rd ed., Oxford: Blackwell Scientific); *Diagnosis of Diseases of the Chest* by Fraser and Paré (in four volumes, 1978/1979, Philadelphia: W. B. Saunders); and by *Pulmonary Diseases and Disorders* by Alfred P. Fishman (1980, New York: McGraw-Hill).

It is a pleasure to record my thanks to many friends and colleagues who have so generously helped me in preparation of this book. These include Dr A. C. Douglas, Dr N. W. Horne, Dr P. M. Warren, Dr M. F. Sudlow, Dr A. G. Leitch, Dr A. J. A. Wightman and Dr D. Lamb. Errors remaining are mine. I am also grateful to the Medical Illustration Department of the University of Edinburgh for providing clear figures from my faltering sketches. My thanks also to Mrs L. Clark for typing the manuscript.

*February 1981*                                          DAVID C. FLENLEY

# Anatomy and Physiology of the Airways

Most people breathe through the nose, the passages from the anterior nares to the larynx forming the *upper airway*, where those air passages from the larynx to the alveoli form the *lower airway*.

## The upper airway

The anterior nares, lined with skin, form the narrowest part of the whole airway. The main nasal passage is divided into two by the nasal septum, and this, combined with the convoluted surface of the turbinates, lined with mucus-secreting ciliated cells, and the change in direction of airflow (Fig. 1), ensure that any large particles in the inspired air stream (coarse mode of the atmospheric aerosol, 5–50 $\mu$m diameter particles) are mostly deposited in the nose. The adenoids and tonsils are aggregations of lymphoid tissue, strategically placed to detect any such particles which are antigenic and so may initiate the immune defences of the respiratory tract.

Disease in the upper airway is often related to respiratory problems. These include the common cold, pharyngitis and sore throat (see Chapter 7); allergic rhinitis with bronchial asthma; nasal polyps with aspirin sensitivity; recurrent sinusitis in some cases of bronchiectasis; and finally, nasopharyngeal carcinoma as a cause of apparent haemoptysis. Three other conditions here are of importance in respiratory medicine. Failure to keep food and oral secretions out of the lower airway results in *aspiration pneumonia* (see Chapter 8), a problem which is always possible when disturbances of swallowing or coughing result from interference with innervation of the larynx. Motor laryngeal innervation is through the vagus, the recurrent laryngeal branch supplying most of the intrinsic laryngeal muscles, except for the superior laryngeal constrictor which is supplied by the superior laryngeal vagal branch, which also carries sensory fibres from the larynx. *Hoarseness* may be due either to intrinsic disease of the vocal cords or to interference with laryngeal innervation. Hoarseness lasting for more than two or three weeks needs investigation, as a quarter of such cases result from cervical or thoracic neoplasms,

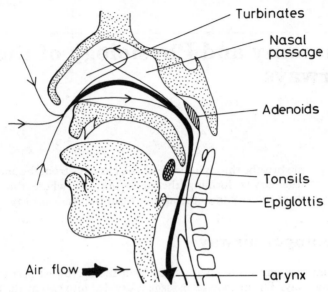

*Fig. 1.*    The upper airway.

particularly secondary spread to the hilar glands from a bronchial carcinoma, interfering with the left recurrent laryngeal nerve as it loops around the left lung hilum. *Obstructive sleep apnoea*, whereby the upper airway becomes intermittently obstructed during sleep, is now recognized to be relatively common in obese adults with a short thick neck, who are heavy snorers (see Chapter 23).

## The lower airway

The lower airway consists of the trachea, two major and 19 segmental bronchi (all with cartilaginous walls), which branch then repeatedly down to the terminal bronchioles, of less than 1 mm in diameter (Fig. 2). These again branch dichotomously into respiratory bronchioles which have some alveoli in their walls, and no longer have ciliated epithelium, and finally to the alveolar ducts and alveolar sacs. The trachea has a diameter of 2.5 cm in the adult, but each lung has some 30 000 terminal bronchioles, each with a diameter of around 0.5 mm. The total cross-sectional area of the lower airway, from the trachea to the alveoli, therefore increases enormously, giving rise to the 'trumpet-shaped' model (Fig. 3). It is obvious that resistance to air flow will thus be greatest in the trachea and major bronchi, where air flow will be most rapid, and much less in the smaller airways, as there

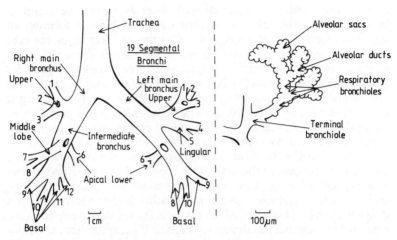

*Fig. 2.*    Branching lower airway. *Left,* trachea and 19 segmental bronchi. *Right,* terminal airway of the respiratory acinus

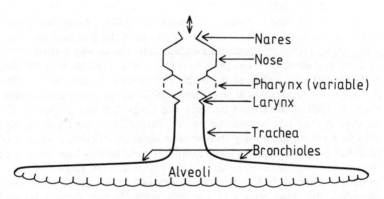

*Fig. 3.*    Cross-sectional area of the airway from the nose to the alveoli (the 'trumpet' model)

are so many of these amongst which the total air flow must be divided, so that flow in these small airways is slow and laminar.

The body has contradictory demands, as the airways should offer a minimal resistance to air flow, and yet minimal dead space (or wasted ventilation). Smooth muscle in the airways, which can thus vary their calibre, may serve to optimize these conflicting demands. The lower airways are lined with ciliated epithelium as far as the terminal bronchi, these cilia and the overlying mucous blanket forming an important defence of the lungs (see Chapter 2). Beating of the cilia moves the overlying mucous blanket continuously from the distal airways towards the tracheal carina, so carrying upwards particles which may have been deposited in the sticky mucous surface. This mucus also contains *immunoglobulins*, predominantly secretory IgA, and *alveolar macrophages*, phagocytic cells which ingest particles, so defending the lungs against infection and particulate pollution. The mucus is secreted by complex branching submucosal glands in the trachea and major bronchi, these structures extending below the basement membrane of the airways. In more peripheral airways mucus is also secreted by globlet cells interspersed with the ciliated epithelium. Small numbers of neuroepithelial bodies (Kultschitzky's cells) of the APUD system, which may secrete vasoactive peptides, are scattered throughout the airway epithelium. This epithelium also has a sensory nerve supply, consisting of *irritant receptors*, submucosal *rapidly adapting stretch receptors*, and finally the *juxtapulmonary capillary (J) receptors* which are at the alveolar level. All different fibres from these receptors run in the vagus, and this also supplies cholinergic efferent fibres to the bronchial smooth muscles.

Aggregates of lymphoid tissue have recently been described in the submucosa of the airways (*bronchus-associated lymphoid tissue, BALT*), which are similar to Peyer's patches in the gut, and may play a role in secretion of immunoglobulins into the airway lumen.

*Bronchial smooth muscle*, present down to the terminal bronchioles, is associated with cartilage in the bronchial wall. In the trachea, this forms the posterior muscle layer between the horse-shoe cartilagenous rings, as well as the spaces between the rings. Smooth muscle in the airways is tonically contracted in life, under vagal innervation, and may serve instantaneously to optimize these conflicting demands of minimal airways resistance and minimal dead space. Contraction of the smooth muscle narrows the airway and is a major feature of many asthmatic attacks. In the asthmatic, airway smooth muscle is hypertrophied; this also occurs in patients with chronic bronchitis and emphysema. Airway smooth muscle possesses $\beta_2$ adrenergic receptors, with the result that sympathomimetic agents induce bronchodilatation. The muscle contracts directly reflexly when the subject inhales histamine and reflex bronchoconstriction also results from stimulation of irritant airway receptors. The airway smooth muscle also contracts in response to prostaglandin $F_{2\alpha}$. Sensitivity to all these bronchoconstrictors (inhaled histamine, prostaglandins and reflex mediated irritants) is greatly increased in asthmatics, who thus display *bronchial hyper-reactivity (or 'twitchy airways')*. The asthmatic attack ensues when such a subject encounters a trigger to the attack, be it of irritant, allergic or occupational origin.

# Measurement of airway calibre

The maximal rate at which air can be blown from the lungs following a vital capacity breath (*peak expiratory flow, PEF*) depends on the mechanical properties of the lungs, including the static elastic recoil pressure (see later) and the diameter of the airways of the lower respiratory tract. However, further muscular effort will not increase the peak flow rate, as this is limited by these intrinsic mechanical properties of the lungs and lower airways. Measurements of PEF made by the Wright peak flow meter are widely used to assess airway calibre in practice. In a normal adult PEF is over 400 litres/minute, but this can fall to as low as 50 litres/minute in an attack of asthma or in a patient with severe chronic bronchitis and emphysema. Recording the volume of air expired in such a maximal expiratory effort, starting from maximal inspiration (total lung capacity), gives the *forced expiratory volume in one second* ($FEV_1$), which is an accurate and reproducible measurement of airway calibre, also very useful in practice. Continuing to blow out until all the air that can be is expelled yields the forced vital capacity (FVC). The ratio of $FEV_1/FVC$ is normally over 70% in health. Obviously small lungs do not hold as much air as large lungs, but presenting results as both the $FEV_1$ and the ratio $FEV_1/FVC$ corrects for this effect. These spirometric measurements are made with the patient exhorted to blow his hardest, following a full inspiration, into a light-weight, water-sealed or bellows spirometer, with a record of expired volume against time (Fig. 4).

An alternative expression of the same information is to plot the instantaneous flow rate during the maximal expiratory blow against the lung volume at which that flow rate occurs, yielding the *flow–volume curve*, from which the peak flow, $FEV_1$ and FVC may be recorded, provided the spirogram against time is also obtained simultaneously. Flow–volume curves can yield more information, as the curve is scalloped downwards towards the volume axis in obstructive lung disease, whereas this descending limb of the curve is relatively straight in health (Fig. 5).

Measurements which do not depend upon maximal expiratory flow can relate airways resistance (measuring during panting in the body plethysmograph, so keeping the larynx fully opened), to the lung volume. As the airways are tethered by the lung parenchyma to the pleura, it is obvious that when the lung volume increases with a full inspiration, the airways will also enlarge in calibre, whereas as when the lung volume falls, the airways will narrow (Fig. 6). Thus, *airways resistance (Raw)* is low at high lung volumes, but increases at low lung volumes (Fig. 6). The relationship is hyperbolic and thus can be linearized by expressing the airways resistance (Raw) as its reciprocal (or *airways conductance, Gaw*), so that the plot of Gaw against lung

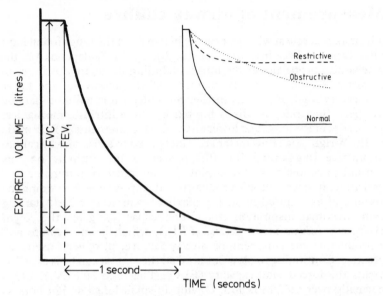

*Fig. 4.*    A forced expiratory spirogram, showing the expired volume against
time during a forced expiration. The FVC is the maximal volume
expired, irrespective of time, whereas the $FEV_1$ is the volume
expired within the first second of the maximal effort from full
inspiration. The inset shows patterns in restriction and obstruction
as opposed to normal

volume is a straight line usually passing through the origin. The slope
of this line is used to determine airways calibre, irrespective of the lung
volume, by the measurement known as the *specific airways conductance*
($S_{Gaw}$).

# Lung volumes

The volume of air within the lungs at maximal inspiration is the total
lung capacity (TLC). If after this maximal inspiration the subject
breathes out as far as he can, the volume of gas expelled from the lungs
is the vital capacity (VC). However, at the end of this maximal
expiration, some gas remains in the lungs which cannot be breathed
out, and this is the residual volume (RV) (Fig. 7).

All these values are measured by simple spirometry, with a dilution
method to measure the RV. Clearly these values vary with size, but
normal values are established for defined age, sex and height. Lung
volumes are altered in many lung diseases. Two characteristic patterns
are described. The first, the *obstructive pattern*, is a combination of

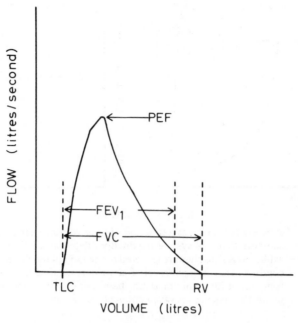

*Fig. 5.*  The flow–volume curve at maximal expiratory flow plotted against lung volume simultaneously recorded. Peak expiratory flow (PEF), $FEV_1$ and FVC are shown. Maximal inspiration is at total lung capacity (TLC), and maximal expiration at residual volume (RV)

increased airways resistance (shown as diminished peak flow, $FEV_1$ and a low $FEV_1/FVC$ ratio, as well as an increased $S_{Gaw}$), coupled with hyperinflation, TLC being above the predicted normal value, and a marked increase in RV, so that the ratio RV/TLC is much above the normal value of around 30% (Fig. 7). This obstructive pattern is characteristic of patients with chronic bronchitis and emphysema and also occurs during an attack of bronchial asthma. The converse, the *restrictive pattern*, has a relatively normal airways resistance ($S_{Gaw}$), as shown by the normal peak flow, normal or slightly low $FEV_1$, but a normal $FEV_1/FVC$ ratio; yet a reduction in TLC, VC and RV (Fig. 7). This restrictive pattern is characteristic of patients with fibrosing and allergic alveolitis, or with space-occupying lesions within the thorax.

# Lung acini and lobules

The business of the lungs is gas exchange, and this occurs in the alveoli, which are contained within the basic anatomical units of the

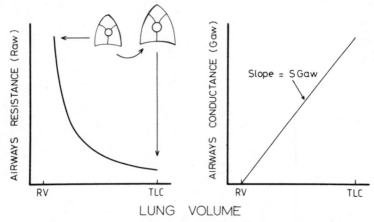

*Fig. 6.*    Airways resistance as a function of lung volume (left-hand panel), showing that airways are maximally dilated at TLC, and smaller calibre at RV, as they are tethered to the lung parenchyma. Airways conductance (the reciprocal of airways resistance) is thus a linear function of lung volume (right-hand panel), the slope of this line being the specific airways conductance (SGaw)

lungs, the acini and lobules. The acinus is supplied by a terminal bronchiole and is the smallest unit of the lung to be surrounded by more or less distinct fibrous septum, the whole acinus measuring about 1 cm in diameter. Some 30–50 lobules form each acinus, each lobule (Fig. 8) being supplied by a respiratory bronchiole, which branches many times into the alveolar ducts and alveoli, there being some 300 million alveoli in each normal adult human lung. The respiratory bronchiole is accompanied into the lobule by a pulmonary arteriole, but the pulmonary venules taking oxygenated blood back from the lobule run in the periphery, towards the incomplete fibrous septa surrounding the acini. The lobules are also drained by pulmonary lymphatics, which drain towards the hilar nodes.

## The alveoli

Gas and blood meet in the alveoli. The pulmonary capillaries are probably not tubular vessels, but more lake-like structures interposed between the air spaces of adjacent alveoli. The final barrier to diffusion of gas from alveoli to the haemoglobin in the red cells consists of (Fig. 9):

1. *The alveolar epithelium,* formed by type I alveolar pneumocytes, disc-like cells which are lined on their alveolar surface by *surfactant.*

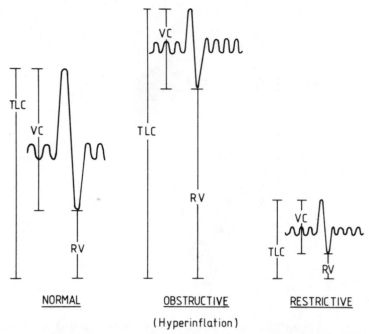

NORMAL          OBSTRUCTIVE          RESTRICTIVE

(Hyperinflation)

*Fig. 7.*   Spirograms of lung volume against time with the subdivisions of volumes in a normal subject, a patient with an obstructive defect with hyperinflation of the lungs, and a patient with a restrictive defect. TLC=total lung capacity; VC=vital capacity; RV= residual volume

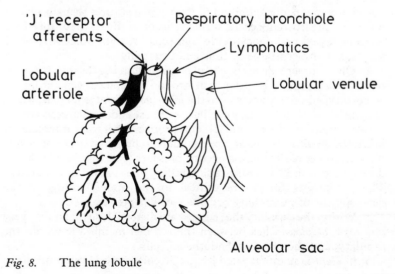

*Fig. 8.*   The lung lobule

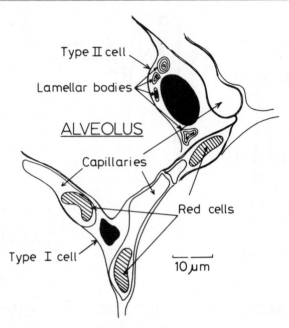

*Fig. 9.*    The alveolar capillary membrane, showing type II alveolar pneumocytes (or 'corner' cells), whose lamellar bodies release surfactant, and alveolar type I pneumocytes, whose thin processes
form the alveolar epithelium. From an electron micrograph

This is a complex phospholipid protein which ensures that alveoli stay
open, as it greatly reduces the surface tension of the air tissue interface.
Alveolar type I pneumocytes are connected by tight junctions, which
are usually impermeable to fluids and proteins.

2. On the inner side of the alveolar epithelium lies the *interstitium of
the alveolar space*, a thin layer of ground substance, separating the
alveolar type I pneumocyte from the *pulmonary endothelial cells*, which
line the lake-like pulmonary capillaries. These endothelial cells are not
joined by tight junctions, and it seems probable that these intercellular
junctions do allow water and crystalloids to pass under the opposing
physical forces of the plasma oncotic pressure (sucking fluid back into
the capillary), and the hydrostatic capillary pressure driving fluid out.
These opposing forces are critical to the understanding of the
development of pulmonary oedema (see Chapter 22).

3. Within the capillary the red cells are distorted, so that only a very
*thin layer of plasma* lies between the red cell membrane within the
capillary, and the capillary endothelial cells.

*Surfactant* is manufactured by the alveolar type II pneumocyte, a

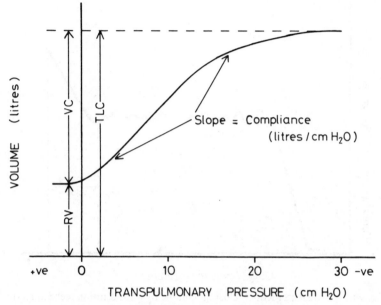

*Fig. 10.*    Static pressure–volume curve of the lungs as the relationship between lung volume from TLC to RV, against transpulmonary pressure. The slope of this line, which varies with the lung volume at which it is measured, is the lung compliance

large cuboidal cell lying in the corners of alveoli, which contains lamellar bodies, probably the origin of the surfactant.

## Lung mechanics

Air is drawn into the chest by descent of the diaphragm and expansion of the rib cage by contraction of the inspiratory muscles. The negative intrapleural pressure thus created distends the lungs by stretching their elastic structures, increasing the volume of the air spaces, so that air rushes in. The relationship between the distending or transpulmonary pressure (measured by a balloon in the lower oesophagus) and the volume of air within the lungs is described by the *static pressure–volume curve of the lungs* (Fig. 10). This curve is sigmoid, as can be easily shown on oneself by first taking in a small breath, from a normal resting breathing position, and then attempting to take the same size of breath in when the lungs are almost filled by a preceding large breath held within the chest. This latter breath is much more difficult to take than the first, showing that the pressure needed to suck in this further

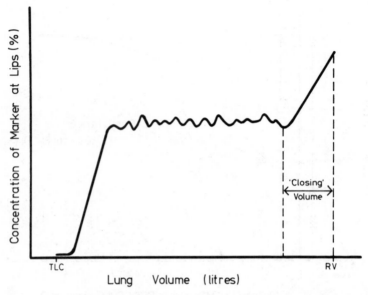

*Fig. 11.*    Measurement of 'closing' volume by a gas dilution technique, the sudden rise in concentration of the marker gas at the lips in a slow expiration indicating the volume of gas left within the lungs at which small airways tend to close. This is the 'closing' volume and maybe increased in small airways disease

volume is much greater than that when the lungs are only slightly filled. At the lower end of the pressure–volume curve it appears that decreasing the transpulmonary pressure, or indeed making it positive, does not cause all the air to be expelled from the chest. The air left behind is the residual volume (RV), trapped behind airways which close at these low transpulmonary pressures. The lung volume at which this closure begins can be measured by an ingenious dilution technique, without measuring transpulmonary pressure, and is known as the *closing volume*, which is increased in disease of the small airways (Fig. 11). However, the hope that this simple physiological test could lead to early detection of such disease in this otherwise 'silent zone' of the lung has not been borne out, as measurements of closing volume are poorly reproducible.

The slope of the pressure–volume curve of the lung defines the amount of pressure required to suck a given amount of gas into them, this value being known as the *lung compliance* or stiffness of the lung. However, it is apparent that the value of lung compliance will depend upon where in the lung volume the measurement is made, as the pressure–volume curve has a sigmoid shape (Fig. 10). Thus, quoting

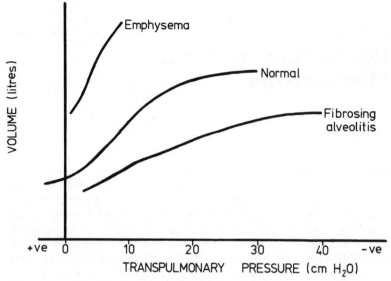

*Fig. 12.*      Changes in static pressure–volume curves of the lungs in emphysema and fibrosing alveolitis, compared to those in the normal subject

single values for lung compliance is useless, whereas measurement and display of the whole pressure–volume curve can be valuable in diagnosis. Thus in chronic bronchitis and emphysema the lungs lose elastic tissue and appear to be very compliant, whereas in fibrosing alveolitis the lungs appear to be very stiff, with a low compliance (Fig. 12).

## Further reading

BATES, D. V., MACKLEM, P. T. and CHRISTIE, R. V. (1971) *Respiratory Function in Disease.* Philadelphia: W. B. Saunders.

BRAIN, J. D., PROCTOR, D. F. and REID, L. M. (1977) *Lung Biology in Health and Disease, Vol. 5, Respiratory Defence Mechanisms, Part 1.* New York: Marcel Dekker.

COTES, J. E. (1975) *Lung Function, Assessment and Application in Medicine,* 3rd ed. Oxford: Blackwell Scientific.

FENN, W. O. and RAHN, H. (1964) *Handbook of Physiology, Section 3, Respiration,* vol. 1. Washington, D.C.: American Physiological Society.

LICHTENSTEIN, L. M. and AUSTEN, K. F. (1977) *Asthma: Physiology, Immunopharmacology and Treatment.* New York: Academic Press.

NADEL, J. A. (1980) *Lung Biology in Health and Disease, vol. 15, Physiology and Pharmacology of the Airways.* New York: Marcel Dekker.

SADOUL, P., MILIC-EMILI, J., SIMONSSON, B. G. and CLARK, T. J. H. (1979) *Small Airways in Health and Disease.* Amsterdam: Excerpta Medica.

SCADDING, J. G., CUMMING, G. and THURLBECK, W. M. (1981) *Scientific Foundations of Respiratory Medicine.* London: Heinemann Medical.

# 2

# Respiratory Defence Mechanisms

The average adult breaths 10 000–20 000 litres (or 15 kg) of atmospheric air each day. This is some ten times more by weight than the amount of either food or water that he uses in a day, showing the great potential of exposure to environmental hazards encountered by the respiratory system. Air contains a variety of potentially harmful agents; particles (forming the atmospheric aerosol), which are of both biological origin (pollens, spores, both bacterial and fungal, bacteria and viruses), as well as chemical and physical particles; in addition to gases and vapours, radioactive substances and ions.

*Atmospheric particles* tend to fall into two size distributions, the *fine mode*, ranging from 0.1 to 1.0 $\mu$m in diameter, and *coarse mode* from 2 to 50 $\mu$m. Fine mode particles are mainly water-soluble and arise from fuel combustion, photochemical oxidation and gas to particle conversion, and consist of sulphates, nitrates, hydrocarbons, carbon and heavy metals, particularly lead and arsenic. Coarse mode particles are less water-soluble, and arise from wind-blown dust and industrial grinding processes. They include silicates, carbonates, ferric oxides, magnesium and calcium ions and pollens. Biological particles occur in both modes, ranging in size from 10 to 100 $\mu$m for pollen grains, 0.3 to 30 $\mu$m for bacteria and 0.03 to 0.05 $\mu$m for viruses.

The *water content of air*, or humidity, varies enormously with climate and temperature, the *relative humidity* being the ratio of the actual water content of an air sample to that when the sample is fully saturated. The optimal humidity at room temperature is from 30 to 60%, but if the nasal airway is bypassed, as with an endotracheal tube, the inspired air must then be nearly 90% saturated. The saturated water vapour pressure ($P\text{H}_2\text{O}$) depends on the temperature; at 37°C $P\text{H}_2\text{O}$ is 6.3 kPa (47 mmHg). The nose is the main site for warming and humidifying the inspired air, but also regains some heat and water vapour from the expired air. A normal man in a temperate climate therefore loses 300–400 ml of water each 24 hours in this respiratory air conditioning. Mouth breathing is much less effective for this purpose, and an 'artificial nose', which ensures precipitation of water from expired air, which can then be picked up again during the ensuing inspiration, is widely used for patients with a tracheostomy.

*Gases in the air* include, of course, nitrogen (78%), oxygen (21%), argon (0.9%) and carbon dioxide (0.03%). Common pollutants in city air include carbon monoxide, sulphur dioxide, nitric and other oxides of nitrogen, but also a host of other potential pollutants, such as hydrogen sulphide, ammonia, sulphuric acid, traces of many metals, and carcinogens such as 3,4-benzpyrene. *Photochemical oxidants* arise from atmospheric interaction between hydrocarbons and nitrogen oxides in sunlight, which forms ozone, peroxylacetyl nitrates and aldehydes, all of which cause irritation of the eyes and respiratory tract, with bronchoconstriction.

# Defence mechanisms

It is clear that human survival is dependent upon the evolution of mechanisms for protecting the respiratory tract against these potential hazards, yet allowing the extraction of sufficient oxygen to sustain life. Breakdown in one or other of these defence mechanisms is a major source of respiratory disease. The defences are the mucociliary blanket, the cough mechanism and cellular and immunological mechanisms.

## The mucociliary blanket

The mucociliary blanket is the major mechanism for clearing particles from the airways surface. It consists of (Fig. 13):

1. A viscid or gel mucus layer containing large glycoprotein molecules which are secreted by goblet cells and submucosal bronchial glands.

2. A water or sol periciliary layer, in which the cilia beat, only their tips projecting into the mucus layer, as relaxation occurs in this watery periciliary layer (Fig. 13). The epithelial basal cells bearing microvilli are involved in production and absorption of this watery layer.

3. The respiratory cilia, some 200/cell, beat towards the mouth at 20 beats/second. Each cilium is 5–50 $\mu$m long, with a complex internal structure of sliding tubules, some components of these, the dynein arms, being missing in the immotile cilia syndrome (see Chapter 12). In health the mucus layer in man moves at about 20 mm/minute, but this is reduced ten-fold in patients with chronic bronchitis and emphysema.

Particles are deposited on the mucociliary blanket by *impaction*, occurring particularly at branches in the airways, *gravitational sedimentation* and *brownian movement*. Particles in the coarse mode of the atmospheric aerosol (2–50 $\mu$m diameter) tend to be deposited in the nasopharynx, only fine mode (0.1–1.0 $\mu$m diameter) particles being deposited in the alveoli. However, particles in this size range may

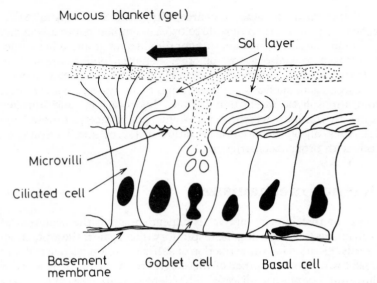

*Fig. 13.*    Cells defining the ciliated respiratory epithelium and the muco-ciliary blanket

undergo *hygroscopic growth*, with an increase in size from absorption of water within the airways; the increase in diameter then also increases their chance of being deposited in alveoli of small airways.

The rate of mucociliary clearance varies in health, being reduced during sleep and in chronic cigarette smokers, but increased in exercise, and following acute exposure to bronchial irritants (tobacco smoke, sulphur dioxide, etc.). Patients with bronchial asthma or chronic bronchitis and emphysema have impaired mucociliary clearance, but this is improved by $\beta_2$ sympathomimetics, but not impeded by ipratropium bromide aerosol, despite its other anticholinergic actions.

## Cough

A cough starts with a brief inspiration, followed by sudden closure of the glottis for about 0.1–0.2 seconds, during which expiratory muscle contraction raises the intrathoracic and abdominal pressures to 50–100 mmHg or more. The glottis then opens suddenly, so that there is a rapid expulsion of the gas compressed within the thorax, peak expiratory flows rising to about 12 litres/second or more in health. The sound of the cough results from rapid oscillations of gas and tissues of the upper airways. Lung airways reflexly narrow during a cough, so increasing the linear velocity of the air flow, thus clearing excess secretions from the trachea and bronchi. Glottic closure is not essential for this clearing, however, and *some* patients with long-standing laryngeal palsy can learn to cough effectively enough to clear their secretions.

Cough is initiated either voluntarily or by reflexes arising from irritant receptors in the larynx, trachea and bronchi. Persistent failure of an effective cough can be life-threatening, from aspiration of food, foreign bodies or secretions into the lungs. *Cough failure* can result from:

1. Local airway anaesthesia, or bypassing of the glottis by an endotracheal tube.

2. Central depression, as in coma, general anaesthesia or following depressant drugs (heroin, codeine, methadone, etc.).

3. Neurological disease, affecting either afferents from the irritant cough receptors, as in trauma of the base of the skull (IXth and Xth cranial nerves); or motor fibres (vagal for laryngeal muscles, phrenic for intercostals), or to the abdominal muscles, as in poliomyelitis, syringomyelia, motor neurone disease, etc.

4. Weakness of expiratory muscles, as in myopathies, spinal cord lesions, following muscle relaxant drugs or in myasthenia gravis.

5. Lung disease, by reduction of the maximal expiratory flow rates from loss of elastic recoil and airway obstruction, as in chronic bronchitis and emphysema.

*Cough syncope*, in which a paroxysm of coughing terminates in an abrupt but transient loss of consciousness, without a fit, is a recognized complication of chronic bronchitis and emphysema. Most patients are men who are otherwise relatively vigorous. Loss of consciousness results from a fall in cerebral blood flow following the marked reduction in venous return during the periods of high intra-abdominal and intrathoracic pressures which precede the expulsive phase of the cough. *Micturition syncope* has a similar basis. Both symptoms may only be described in response to a direct question to the patient.

## Cellular and immune defences

Cellular and immune defences are extremely important, for interference with their proper function is a potent source of respiratory disease.

*Pulmonary alveolar macrophages (PAM)*, derived from circulating monocytes, are normal inhabitants of the alveoli and airways. They are motile phagocytic cells which can ingest foreign particles, including micro-organisms. Some micro-organisms are then killed, particularly when the PAM are activated by the lymphokines secreted by T lymphocytes as part of the cellular immune response. Lymphokines include macrophage inhibitory factor (MIF; a glycoprotein of 20 000–40 000 daltons molecular weight), which is released following T cell binding of antigen. Activated macrophages secrete plasminogen activators; proteases, collagenases and elastases (potential causes of emphysema; see Chapter 9); and complement components C2, C3, C4 and C5.

*Polymorphonuclear leucocytes (PMN)* are motile cells, the short-lived circulating phagocytes of the inflammatory response, capable of killing many micro-organisms after phagocytosis by means of the myeloperoxidase–hydrogen peroxide–halide enzyme systems contained within their lysosomes. PMN are drawn from the blood stream to the sites of bacterial invasion by C3a and C5, the chemotactic complement components, and then ingest the bacteria, after binding of the bacterial wall antigen to specific IgG (opsonization).

*B lymphocytes* compromise 5–10% of circulating blood lymphocytes in man, and are responsible for humoral immunity. They multiply and transform into plasma cells after binding of antigen to the specific immunoglobulin receptors carried in their surface. Plasma cells secrete the specific immunoglobulins, IgA, IgC, IgM, IgD and IgE into plasma. Specific antigen-induced proliferation and transformation of a clone of B cells carrying that specific antibody is responsible for the production of immunoglobulins against that specific antigen.

*T lymphocytes*, forming 80–90% of circulating lymphocytes in the blood stream, are responsible for *cell-mediated immunity*, and also interact positively with (helper T cells) or inhibit (suppressor T cells) B lymphocytes and macrophages. Cellular immunity underlies delayed hypersensitivity and is particularly important in defence against intracellular pathogens (e.g. *Mycobacterium tuberculosis*), which may not be killed after macrophage phagocytosis alone.

*Complement* consists of a series of 17 plasma proteins, nine in the classical pathway and eight in the alternative pathway, both centering about the proteolytic cleavage of the C3 component (Fig. 14). In the *classical pathway* binding of antigen to antibody (IgG, and particularly IgM) initiates formation of C3 convertase, the resulting C3 cleavage yielding C3b and activating the effector complex C5–C9. In addition the *alternative pathway* amplification C3 convertase (C3b, Bb) is assembled on the surface of an appropriate initiating agent. The alternative pathway can also be triggered directly by the cell surfaces of micro-organisms which lack surface sialic acid, without prior antigen–antibody binding. The effector complex C5–C9 results from activation of either pathway, and it can kill cells directly. Smaller cleavage products of C3 (C3a) and later components (C5a) are anaphylatoxins causing vasodilatation and attract PMN.

*Immunoglobulins*, synthesized by plasma cells, are circulating plasma proteins which bind specific antigen. *IgM* is usually confined to the blood stream by its large size (900 000 daltons) and is the earliest specific antibody produced in response to an antigen, with a half life of some five days, and a plasma concentration of 100 mg/dl. IgM binds antigen

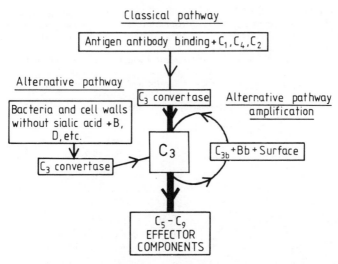

*Fig. 14.*    Components and interactions of the complement pathway

very effectively, with activation of complement. *IgG* has a plasma concentration of about 1000 mg/dl, with a molecular weight of 156 000 daltons, and is thus found in some extravascular fluids, IgG also activates complement. *IgA* (150 000–350 000 daltons) has a plasma concentration of 250 mg/dl, but also includes *secretory IgA*, which is found in respiratory tract secretions, but does not there activate complement, although inactivating virus particles. *IgE*, present in the very low concentration of only 0.01 mg/dl in plasma, has a molecular weight of 190 000 daltons. It binds specific antigen to mast cells, with release of anaphylatoxins (histamine, serotonin, ECF-A, SRS-A, etc.) and is present in increased concentrations in the serum of atopic subjects, and in those with intestinal helminth infestations.

*Interferon* consists of three species-specific proteins of about 30 000 daltons in man. Synthesis of the interferons can be provoked in cells by viral infection (foreign double-stranded RNA), as well as by synthetic interferon inducers (e.g. anionic polymers and polynucleotides) and bacterial endotoxin. Interferon acts on adjacent cells in the respiratory epithelium to inhibit further replication of viral messenger RNA for some 24 hours. However, 20 years after its discovery, interferon has not so far been found a role in the therapy of viral respiratory infections in man.

## Further reading

BENACERRAF, B. and UNANUE, E. R. (1979) *Textbook of Immunology.* Baltimore: Williams & Wilkins.

BRAIN, J. D., PROCTOR, D. F. and REID, L. M. (1977) *Lung Biology in Health and Disease, vol. 5, Respiratory Defence Mechanisms, Part II*. New York: Marcel Dekker.

BRAIN, J. D. and VALBERG, P. A. (1979) Deposition of aerosol in the respiratory tract. *Am. Rev. resp. Dis.*, **120**, 1325–1374

CAMNER, P. (1980) Clearance of particles from the human tracheobronchial tree. *Clin. Sci.*, **59**, 78–84

NADEL, J. A. (1980) *Lung Biology in Health and Disease, vol. 15, Physiology and Pharmacology of the Airways*. New York: Marcel Dekker.

ROITT, I. (1977) *Essential Immunology*, 3rd ed. Oxford: Blackwell Scientific.

# 3

# Gas Exchange and Acid–Base Balance

## Gas exchange

The respiratory function of the lungs is to add oxygen to the blood and to remove $CO_2$. This is achieved by ventilation of perfused alveoli. The efficiency of gas transfer within an alveolus depends upon the ratio of the alveolar ventilation ($\dot{V}a$) to perfusion ($\dot{Q}$). This $\dot{V}a/\dot{Q}$ ratio varies slightly amongst the 300 million alveoli of the lungs, even in health, but the ratio is very variable in disease, where some alveoli can have a low perfusion, yet a high ventilation (a relative increase in dead space), and yet others poor ventilation but excessive perfusion (relative shunt). The effects of such variabilities on the resultant *arterial blood gas tensions* depend upon the shape of the oxygen and carbon dioxide dissociation curves for blood.

*The oxygen dissociation curve* (*ODC*) relating the *oxygen saturation* ($So_2$) to the oxygen tension ($Po_2$) is sigmoid, as the addition of one molecule of oxygen affects the affinity of the haemoglobin molecule to the next, until all four molecules of oxygen have bound to the haemoglobin, so saturating it. The colour of a blood sample depends upon $So_2$:

$$So_2 = \frac{\text{oxygen concentration at the prevailing } Po_2}{\text{oxygen concentration when fully saturated}}$$

The denominator of this equation, the oxygen concentration when fully saturated, is the oxygen capacity, which in turn depends upon the haemoglobin concentration, as each gram of haemoglobin can bind 1.34 ml of oxygen at 36°C. Thus, although the arterial $So_2$ ($Sao_2$) may be the same in a patient with polycythaemia as in another patient with anaemia, the anaemic patient will carry much less oxygen in each 100 ml of blood.

The shape and position of the ODC depends on the body temperature, and upon concentration of various other small molecules or *ligands*, which can also bind to haemoglobin within the red cell, as well as the oxygen binding. The position of the ODC is defined by the $P_{50}$ ($Po_2$ at 50% $So_2$; Fig. 15). The position of the ODC is abnormal in

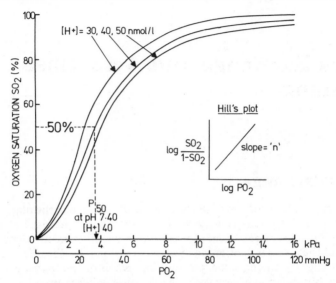

*Fig. 15.*    The oxygen dissociation curve relating oxygen saturation ($SO_2$) to oxygen tension ($PO_2$), showing $P_{50}$, the oxygen tension at one-half full saturation. Three different curves at various levels of acidity [$H^+$] are shown, and the inset shows Hill's plot used to linearize the dissociation curve, and thus shows the slope 'n', which, along with the $P_{50}$, determines the shape and position of the dissociation curve. (*From Flenley 1978*)

many of the *inherited haemoglobinopathies*, where genetic abnormalities in haemoglobin synthesis alter the amino acid sequence in the globin chains. Polycythaemia is common in those haemoglobinopathies with a low $P_{50}$, as for example haemoglobin Chesapeake. The hydrogen ion activity (pH or [$H^+$]) within the red cell is also a major determinant of $P_{50}$ in normal adult haemoglobin, but as this is constantly related to the pH of the plasma, the effect is usually expressed at plasma pH, so that $P_{50}$ is usually defined as being measured at pH 7.4. Acidosis moves the curve to the right (increasing $P_{50}$), whereas alkalosis moves the ODC to the left, with a reduction in $P_{50}$ (Fig. 15). Other ligands of the haemoglobin molecule include 2,3-diphosphoglycerate (2,3-DPG), a byproduct of glycolytic metabolism within the red cell. Blood for transfusion that has been stored in acid citrate dextrose has little DPG, so that such a massive transfusion may interfere with oxygen transport by lowering $P_{50}$ for hours or even days.

*Carbon monoxide* binds much more readily to haemoglobin than does oxygen, but the resultant carboxyhaemoglobin (HbCO) also affects the shape and position of the dissociation curve, as well as preventing oxygen from combining with the haemoglobin already bound as HbCO. Cigarette smoke contains carbon monoxide, so that the HbCO concentration varies from a normal value of less than 2% up to 20% in the heavy cigarette smoker. Although domestic gas now has little carbon monoxide, many deaths in fires result from carbon monoxide poisoning. High concentrations also exist in exhaust fumes of motor cars, so that carbon monoxide poisoning is still an important cause of attempted suicide. *Hyperbaric oxygenation* has been used very effectively to save life in these patients, but the organizational problems of providing this complex and expensive technology at a moment's notice have prevented its widespread adoption. *Carbon monoxide poisoning* needs urgent treatment by administration of as high a concentration of oxygen as possible, combined with hyperventilation of the patient's lungs through a cuffed endotracheal tube. Mouth-to-mouth ventilation with the rescuer's inspired air, as a first-aid measure, has saved many lives and carries no risk to the rescuer.

In a resting healthy subject venous blood perfusing the lungs by the pulmonary artery has a $PO_2$ of 5.3–6.6 kPa (40–50 mmHg), with an $SO_2$ of around 70–80%. The higher partial pressure of oxygen in the ventilated alveolus ($PAO_2$) drives oxygen down its chemical diffusion gradient to the haemoglobin within the red cells in the pulmonary capillaries. In the imaginary 'ideal' alveolus, which is a mathematical abstraction used to describe gas exchange, this alveolar oxygen tension ($PAO_2$) can be approximately derived as:

$$PAO_2 = PIO_2 - \frac{PaCO_2}{R}$$

where $PIO_2$ is the inspired oxygen tension (fractional concentration; $FIO_2$, multiplied by the baromatric pressure minus the vapour pressure of water); $PaCO_2$ is the arterial $PCO_2$; and R the gas exchange ratio, which in most clinical circumstances can be assumed to be 0.8–1.0. At sea level $PIO_2$ is 20 kPa (150 mmHg). The notion behind this simplified form of the *alveolar air equation* is simple; the alveolus contains carbon dioxide evolved from the venous blood and this dilutes the oxygen in the inspired air in the alveolus. The *alveolar to arterial oxygen tension gradient* ($PAO_2 - PaO_2$ or $A - aDO_2$) is thus an indication of the overall efficiency of the lungs in oxygenation, with a value rarely exceeding 2.5 kPa (20 mmHg) in health. If, however, some blood perfuses alveoli which are not ventilated, so forming a venous admixture or 'shunt', this blood will not be oxygenated, and will thus lower the arterial $PO_2$. Such a shunt effect is prominent in many lung diseases, notably in the adult respiratory distress syndrome (see Chapter 11), and is recognized by the small rise in $PaO_2$ which follows

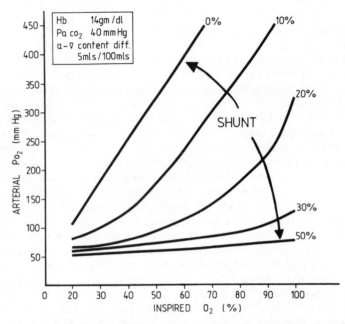

*Fig. 16.*    The relationship between inspired oxygen concentration ($FIO_2$) and arterial oxygen tension ($PaO_2$) at various increasing shunt values. As the shunt fraction increases, arterial $PO_2$ is less influenced by a rise in the inspired oxygen concentration

a large rise in the inspired oxygen concentration (Fig. 16). Clearly, blood which has perfused non-ventilated alveoli will not be exposed to oxygenation no matter what the concentration of the inspired oxygen that is administered to the patient.

In diffusing from the alveolus to the pulmonary capillary, oxygen must traverse various membranes, including the alveolar type I epithelial cell, the interstitial space, the pulmonary endothelial cell, a thin layer of plasma, the red cell membrane and finally combine with the haemoglobin molecule within the red cells (see Fig. 9).

*Arterial hypoxaemia*, with an arterial $PO_2$ below the normal value of 10–12 kPa (75–100 mmHg) is caused by:

1. Reduced $PIO_2$ (inspired oxygen tension), as with high altitude, or from a faulty anaesthetic or respiratory apparatus which delivers a gas with reduced oxygen tension. *Unexpected cyanosis in any patient attached to any breathing system should immediately lead to removal of the system, allowing the patient to breath air, or immediate administration of pure oxygen.*

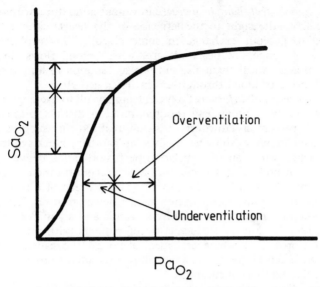

*Fig. 17.*    Overventilation of some alveoli, increased $Po_2$ in blood coming from those alveoli, cannot compensate for underventilation of other alveoli, with a corresponding decrease in $Po_2$, due to the sigmoid shape of the ODC. Clearly the resulting $Sao_2$ from the two sets of alveoli will be lower than if both sets of alveoli had the same ventilation/perfusion ratio

2. *Ventilation/perfusion imbalance,* for overventilation of some perfused alveoli, so raising their $PAo_2$, cannot increase the $So_2$ of the capillary blood coming from these alveoli enough to compensate for a corresponding underventilation (and reduction in $PAo_2$) to other alveoli, where $So_2$ is disproportionately lower. This arises from the sigmoid shape of the oxygen dissociation curve (Fig. 17). However, this mechanism does *not* cause a rise in $Paco_2$, as the carbon dioxide dissociation curve, relating the blood concentration of carbon dioxide to $Pco_2$, is approximately linear over the narrow physiological range, so that here overventilation of some alveoli does indeed compensate for underventilation of other alveoli. Thus, ventilation/perfusion imbalance is by far the commonest cause of hypoxaemia in disease, as in type I respiratory failure (see Chapter 11).

3. *Hypoventilation,* where the arterial $Pco_2$ is raised, indicating that overall alveolar ventilation is inadequate for the metabolic needs of that patient. Hypoventilation may be combined with ventilation/perfusion imbalance, as in type II respiratory failure in patients with chronic bronchitis and emphysema (see Chapter 11).

4. *A physiological shunt*, or increase in venous admixture, with blood passing from the right to the left side of the heart without being exposed to gaseous exchange in some alveoli. This explains the cyanosis of congenital heart disease, where blood flows through abnormal anatomical channels, and is also common in lung disease, with shunting of blood through unventilated alveoli.

5. *Impairment of diffusion* of oxygen from alveoli to haemoglobin in the red cells was previously thought to be a distinct mechanism causing hypoxaemia. However, it is now realized that such patients (previously known as showing an alveolar–capillary block syndrome) have marked variation of ventilation/perfusion ratios between different alveoli, and it is this mechanism which accounts for most of their hypoxaemia. Nonetheless, the physiological pattern of a restrictive defect in lung volumes, combined with a lower transfer factor for carbon monoxide ($T$CO), arterial hypoxaemia and a low $P$CO$_2$ in the arterial blood, remains characteristic of patients with diffuse pulmonary fibrosis, of whatever cause, although the cause of their hypoxaemia can no longer be adequately attributed to thickening of the alveolar capillary membrane.

*Carbon dioxide transport* is also a major function of haemoglobin. Reduced haemoglobin combines with carbon dioxide to form carbamino compounds, but this carbon dioxide is partly displaced as the haemoglobin molecule is oxygenated. Thus, the $P$CO$_2$ of a blood sample rises as the sample is oxygenated, if the oxygenation occurs in a closed system, as in the blood stream. This Christiansen–Douglas–Haldane effect contributes to a small part of the rise in $P$CO$_2$ which often occurs in patients with type II respiratory failure who are given high concentrations of oxygen to breathe. The major carbon dioxide content of the blood is, however, in the bicarbonate ion, both in the plasma and the red cell. The simple equation:

$$\underset{\text{gas}}{CO_2} \rightleftharpoons \underset{\text{solution}}{CO_2} + H_2O \underset{\substack{\text{carbonic} \\ \text{anhydrase}}}{\rightleftharpoons} H_2CO_3 \underset{\substack{\text{ionic} \\ \text{dissoc-} \\ \text{iation}}}{\rightleftharpoons} H^+ + HCO_3^- \qquad (1)$$

is the key to understanding the acid–base balance of the body. The $P$CO$_2$ of mixed venous blood entering the lungs in the pulmonary artery, in a healthy resting subject, is 6.3 kPa (47 mmHg), only 1 kPa (7.5 mmHg) higher than the arterial $P$CO$_2$. Thus, ventilation/perfusion imbalance has much less effect on arterial $P$CO$_2$ than it does upon arterial $P$O$_2$, as a result of this small arteriovenous gradient for $P$CO$_2$. As a result arterial $P$CO$_2$ closely reflects the level of alveolar ventilation. Hyperventilation reduces arterial $P$CO$_2$, and hypoventilation (type II respiratory failure) raises the $P$aCO$_2$. These changes will have corresponding effects upon blood acidity.

# Acid–base balance

The acidity of the blood can be expressed as either the pH, or the hydrogen ion activity $[H^+]$, measured in nanomol/litre. They are related as:

$$pH = \log \frac{1}{[H^+]}$$

The chemical relationships shown in equation (1) can be expressed mathematically by application of the law of mass action to equation (1):

$$[H^+] = \frac{K'_1 \propto PCO_2}{[HCO_3^-]}$$

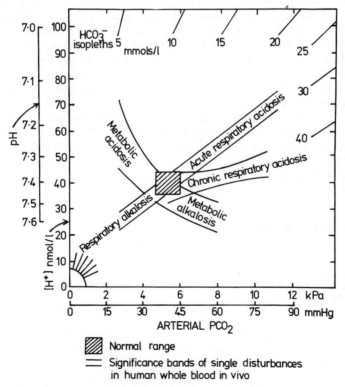

*Fig. 18.*  Acid–base diagram relating blood acidity (pH or $[H^+]$) to arterial $PCO_2$ in the body. (*From Flenley 1978*)

where $K'_1$ is the first dissociation constant of carbonic acid in plasma; $\propto$ is the solubility of $CO_2$ in plasma; $P_{CO_2}$ is arterial $P_{CO_2}$; and $[HCO_3^-]$ is arterial bicarbonate concentration. There must be a linear relationship therefore between $[H^+]$ and $P_{CO_2}$, when both are plotted on non-logarithmic scales, with lines of equal bicarbonate concentration radiating from the origin of such a graph (Fig. 18). This *acid–base diagram* also shows the 95% confidence limits of single clinical disturbances of acid–base balance, as observed in clinical practice in whole arterial blood within the body. In *metabolic acidosis* the primary disturbance is a rise in $[H^+]$ and, as the diagram shows, this increase in acidity stimulates ventilation, so causing a fall in arterial $P_{CO_2}$. Conversely, in *respiratory alkalosis*, hyperventilation causes a fall in $P_{CO_2}$ as the primary disturbance, with resultant fall in $[H^+]$, as dictated by equation (1). A primary rise in $P_{CO_2}$, due to the hypoventilation of type II respiratory failure, causes a corresponding rise in $[H^+]$. If this hypoventilation results acutely, the relationships between $P_{CO_2}$ and $[H^+]$ are those shown in the *acute respiratory acidosis* band on the diagram, whereas if this elevation of $P_{CO_2}$ persists for some days, the renal tubules increase reabsorption of bicarbonate from the tubular fluid, so raising the plasma bicarbonate concentration. As a result the blood becomes less acid, with a fall in $[H^+]$ for the same level of $P_{CO_2}$. The $[H^+]/P_{CO_2}$ relationships now lie within the *chronic respiratory acidosis* band of the diagram. It must be emphasized that these bands are those actually determined in human subjects, and reflect the body's response to these disturbances in acid–base balance. If blood is mixed with gas outside the body, the $[H^+]/P_{CO_2}$ relationships may be somewhat different. As modern blood gas equipment directly measures the $P_{CO_2}$ and $[H^+]$ of blood sampled directly from the artery, these differences, which have caused hot debate between clinical chemists in the past, are of little relevance today to the practising clinician.

## Further reading

FILLEY, G. F. (1971) *Acid and Blood Gas Regulation*. Philadelphia: Lea & Febiger.
FLENLEY, D. C. (1978) Clinical physiology: interpretation of blood gas and acid base data. *Br. J. Hosp. Med.*, **20**, 384–394.
GARBY, L. and MELDON, J. (1977) Respiratory functions of the blood. *Topics in Haematology*. New York and London: Plenum.
WEST, J. B. (1977) *Pulmonary Pathophysiology: The Essentials*. Oxford: Blackwell Scientific.

# 4

# Respiratory Muscles and the Control of Breathing

## Respiratory muscles

Lung ventilation results from repetitive contraction of the inspiratory muscles, which are the diaphragm, intercostal and accessory muscles, and the abdominal muscles. These contractions are under involuntary control, which is adjusted over the long term to meet the body's demands for provision of oxygen and removal of carbon dioxide, so that the arterial blood gas tensions are kept within close limits ($PO_2$ 10–12 kPa, 70–100 mmHg; $PCO_2$ 4.6–6.0 kPa, 35–45 mmHg) in health. This involuntary control can be temporarily over-riden by voluntary contractions, as in speech, and is influenced by reflexes, from irritant receptors in the nose and upper airway (cough and sneeze), by vagal afferents from the lung (airway irritant receptors, stretch receptors and 'J' receptors), and by somatic afferents from muscle and skin.

The *respiratory muscles* are skeletal-striated muscles. The diaphragm is the most important inspiratory muscle and may be the only muscle effectively contracting during quiet breathing in upright man. Diaphragmatic contraction displaces the abdomen outward, lifting and expanding the rib cage, so creating the negative intrapleural pressure which inflates the lungs. This negative intrapleural pressure would tend to draw the lower rib cage inward, were it not opposed by inspiratory contraction of the intercostal muscles. Abdominal muscle contraction improves the mechanical advantage of the diaphragm by increasing the abdominal pressure, so raising and thus stretching the diaphragm, and thus making its contraction more efficient (Fig. 19).

*Diaphragmatic paralysis*, when unilateral, causes few symptoms. Phrenic nerve involvement by tumour at the hilum of the lung is the commonest cause. Diaphragmatic screening, whereby a sniff induces a paradoxical upward movement of more than 2 cm in the paralysed diaphragm is diagnostic of unilateral diaphragmatic paralysis. Rarer causes include pneumonia, neck trauma and herpes zoster, but sometimes the cause is never found, and in many of these cases the paralysis improves spontaneously. Bilateral diaphragmatic paralysis is rare, but can follow neck trauma, infections and myopathies. Severe breathlessness results, the vital capacity (VC) being reduced by up to

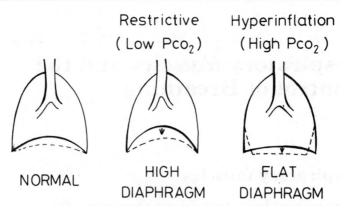

*Fig. 19.*    Effect of position of the diaphragm at the end of expiration (solid line) on the contraction achieved by the end of inspiration (dotted line) in normal subjects, restrictive defect with a high diaphragm, and in hyperinflation with a low flat diaphragm

50%, and the breathlessness is often worse when lying down. A paradoxical inward movement of the abdominal wall on inspiration in the supine patient is a useful clinical sign of bilateral diaphragmatic paralysis. These patients are usually hypoxic when lying supine, and this can be greatly exaggerated during sleep.

*Diaphragmatic hernia* can occur through the oesophageal hiatus (hiatus hernia), and less commonly through the foramen of Morgagni (which can be confused radiologically with a pleuropericardial cyst), or posterolaterally through the foramen of Bochdalek, which can be a cause of respiratory distress in the neonate.

*Hiccup* is an intermittent voluntary contraction of the diaphragm, often unilaterally on the left side. It can occur in meningitis, brain tumour, uraemia, gastrointestinal disorders, including gastric dilatation, and pancreatic disease. Remedies for persistent hiccup vary from a drink of cold water, via phenothiazines, to a phrenic nerve crush, the latter only being contemplated in severe, protracted, and otherwise intractable cases.

*Diaphragmatic fatigue,* along with fatigue of other inspiratory muscles, has now become recognized as a potential cause of respiratory failure. Fatigue can be induced experimentally in man. In a patient with hyperinflation of the chest, and thus a low and flattened diaphragm, the association of inward abdominal motion with outward rib cage expansion occurring during inspiration (*Hoover's sign*) is thought to represent an ineffective diaphragmatiç contraction. The sign appears to carry a bad prognosis in a patient with chronic bronchitis and emphysema, if seen during an acute exacerbation of the disease. A sophisticated analysis of the EMG has recently been

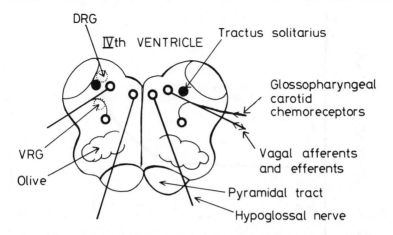

DRG

IVth VENTRICLE

Tractus solitarius

Glossopharyngeal
carotid
chemoreceptors

VRG

Olive

Vagal afferents
and efferents

Pyramidal tract

Hypoglossal nerve

*Fig. 20.*    Probable arrangement of respiratory centres — dorsal respiratory group (DRG) and ventral respiratory group (VRG) — in the brain stem of man, based upon actual physiological studies in the cat

claimed to enable the diagnosis of respiratory muscle fatigue to be made at an earlier stage, but this work is still controversial.

Other causes of respiratory muscle fatigue include obesity, neuro-muscular disorders (including hemiplegia) and severe kyphoscoliosis.

## The neural control of breathing

Recent neurological studies in animals have led to the re-establishment of the concept of the respiratory centres in the medulla oblongata, with description of a dorsal respiratory group (DRG) lying near to the nucleus of the tractus solitarius, and a ventral respiratory group (VRG) which is related to the vagal motor fibres (Fig. 20). A flip–flop activation of inspiratory neurones alternating with expiratory activity, is generated in small interneurones known as paired pattern generators. These are in turn primarily driven by the afferent inputs from the carotid body and central (medullary) carbon dioxide chemoreceptors. Vagal sensory fibres, serving to inhibit inspiration on distension of the lungs (Hering-Breuer reflex), act on the DRG and central pattern generator, whereas the VRG group provide stimulation to both phrenic and intercostal motor neurones, and also to vagal motor fibres.

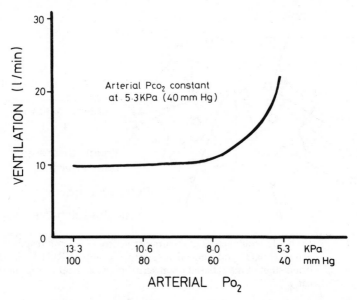

*Fig. 21.*    The relationship between minute ventilation and arterial $P_{O_2}$ as $P_{O_2}$ is progressively lowered experimentally in a normal subject, yet maintaining arterial $P_{CO_2}$ constant at normal values. Note that ventilation does not increase until the $P_{O_2}$ falls below 8.0 kPa (60 mmHg)

## Chemoreceptors

Arterial hypoxaemia, if sufficiently severe ($P_{O_2}$ less than 8.0 kPa, 60 mmHg), stimulates ventilation progressively as the hypoxaemia becomes more severe (Fig. 21) if the $P_{CO_2}$ is kept unchanged. This stimulation arises from the chemoreceptors in the carotid body, a small structure some 1.3 mm in diameter, situated at the bifurcation of the carotid arteries. The carotid body has a very rich blood supply, and a complex sensory system, with intercalated neurones, sensitive to dopamine and noradrenaline as neurotransmitters. The afferent nerve fibres from the carotid body run in a branch of the glossopharyngeal nerve to the medulla. The carotid body also responds to arterial acidity and raised $P_{CO_2}$, as well as its major response to hypoxia. Chronic hypoxia, as in people living at high altitude and patients with chronic bronchitis and emphysema, is associated with enormous hypertrophy of the carotid body, to some ten times its normal weight. The cause and mechanism of this hypertrophy are not fully understood.

Central chemoreceptors on the lateral border of the medulla are sensitive to the acidity of the bathing cerebrospinal fluid. The central

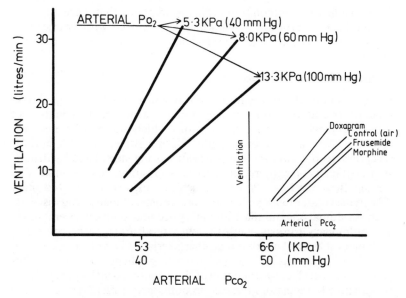

Fig. 22. The relationship between minute ventilation and arterial $PCO_2$ at three different levels of arterial $PO_2$, showing the interaction between these two chemical stimuli in controlling ventilation. The inset shows the effects of drugs on this relationship, at normal arterial $PO_2$. Note that doxapram (the respiratory stimulant) increases sensitivity to carbon dioxide, whereas frusemide and morphine both reduce this sensitivity in a normal subject

chemoreceptors thus serve the ventilatory response to carbon dioxide, which stimulates ventilation by causing the CSF to become more acid, and so stimulating the central chemoreceptors. In normal man hypoxia and a raised $PCO_2$ interact to drive ventilation (Fig. 22). Chemical control mechanisms seem to provide the long-term stability of the ventilatory drive, so ensuring that arterial blood gas tensions remain constant.

Many drugs affect the chemical drive to breathing. Narcotic analgesics (heroin, morphine, pethidine, methadone, and probably codeine) also depress the ventilatory response to both hypoxia and carbon dioxide. Hypnotics share a similar action, particularly with all barbiturates, but also the widely used non-barbiturate hypnotics, nitrazepam and flurazepam, can also depress ventilatory response to carbon dioxide, particularly in patients with carbon dioxide retention, as in type II respiratory failure in chronic bronchitis and emphysema. Similar actions have been documented with diazepam and chlordiazepoxide, the common tranquillizers, implying that there is no safe tranquillizer or hypnotic agent which can be used with impunity in patients with carbon dioxide retention.

## Vagal afferent fibres

Receptors in the lungs are important in controlling breathing. These include irritant receptors in the bronchi, which cause cough, and bronchoconstriction; stretch receptors which inhibit the next inspiration after a deep breath (the Hering-Breuer reflex), and 'J' receptors deep within the lungs possibly being stimulated by distension of the alveolar interstitial space, as in pulmonary oedema. The Hering-Breuer reflex is not demonstrable in unanaesthetized man. The hyperventilation which is so characteristic of many lung diseases, such as asthma, pneumonia, pulmonary oedema, pulmonary embolism and pulmonary fibrosis, causes a low arterial $P\text{CO}_2$ to be combined with modest arterial hypoxaemia, characteristically with an increase in the alveolar to arterial oxygen tension gradient $(\text{A–a}D\text{O}_2)$. This probably results from stimulation of 'J' receptors, which appear also to be sensitive to mediators released in pulmonary inflammation, or the asthmatic attack. Such hyperventilation clearly cannot arise from a central chemoreceptor drive, as the low arterial $P\text{CO}_2$ would switch off such a drive.

# Exercise

The hyperventilation of exercise remains a physiological mystery, but current theories propose that this depends upon the increased transport of carbon dioxide to the lungs from the exercising muscles, the increase in ventilation being sufficient to maintain the arterial $P\text{CO}_2$ constant. The carotid bodies play some role in this mechanism, for their surgical removal (a very controversial Californian treatment for asthma) delays the rate at which the ventilation increases at the start of exercise. Neural inputs from the exercising muscles also play some role in exercise hyperventilation.

In *exercise tests* the minute ventilation $(\dot{V}\text{E})$ is related to the measured oxygen consumption $(\dot{V}\text{O}_2)$ during a progressive increase in the work load, usually during bicycle exercise. Excessive ventilation for a given oxygen consumption is characteristic of diffuse lung diseases (fibrosing and allergic alveolitis, stage II or III sarcoidosis, pulmonary thromboembolic disease, etc.), and in these conditions the arterial oxygen saturation $(Sa\text{O}_2)$ and $P\text{O}_2$ will often also fall as the level of exercise increases, even although the values were normal when at rest. This fall in $Sa\text{O}_2$ is not a feature of psychogenic hyperventilation on exercise. Measurement of $\text{FEV}_1$ before, during and after exercise may give clear objective evidence of exercised-induced asthma, very characteristic of atopic asthma. In more disabled patients, who tolerate mouth-pieces and other measuring equipment poorly, useful assessment can be obtained by measuring the distance that they walk, at their own pace, within a 12-minute period on a level surface.

# Breathlessness

Breathlessness is a symptom and not a sign. However, there is still lacking a firm physiological explanation of the sensation, which is usually agreed to be an unpleasant sensation related to an increased demand for breathing, and appears to relate to disproportion between the physiological demand and the actual ventilation which is generated. Breathlessness is only rarely a primary result of hypoxaemia in disease, particularly when the breathlessness is present at rest, but more usually originates from other mechanisms related to the cause of the hypoxaemia, as in widespread lung disease.

## Further reading

DERENNE, J. P., MACKLEM, P. T. and ROUSSOS, C. (1978) The respiratory muscles: mechanics, control and pathophysiology, parts I–III. *Am. Rev. resp. Dis.*, **118**, 119–134, 373–390, 581–602.
INTERNATIONAL SYMPOSIUM ON THE DIAPHRAGM (1979) *Am. Rev. resp. Dis.*, **19**, Suppl. 1–181.
SAUNDERS, K. B. (1977) *Clinical Physiology of the Lung*. Oxford: Blackwell Scientific.
WILLIAMS, M. H. (1980) *Clinics in Chest Medicine, 1. Disturbance of Respiratory Control*. Philadelphia: W. B. Saunders.

# 5

# Symptoms and Signs of Respiratory Disease

## Symptoms

There are six common symptoms of respiratory disease; cough, sputum, haemoptysis, breathlessness, wheeze and chest pain.

### Cough

Cough can be dry (or non-productive) or with production of sputum. A persistent cough is abnormal. A heavy smoker may fail to recognize this, whereas his 'normal smoker's cough' is, in fact, a sign of hypersecretion of mucus leading to his impending or actual chronic bronchitis.

*Recurrent dry cough* may be due to:
1. The early stage of tracheal or lung infection, notably virus pneumonia, or pulmonary tuberculosis.
2. Impending left heart failure, where the cough characteristically wakes the patient from sleep.
3. Bronchial carcinoma, where cough is characteristically an early symptom.
4. A nervous habit, which is of no clinical significance.

*Productive cough* can be due to:
1. Pneumonia, of viral, bacterial (including tuberculosis), mycotic, rickettsial or parasitic origin.
2. Irritation from noxious gases, smoke or foreign bodies.
3. Allergy as in asthma or allergic rhinitis.
4. Neoplasm, particularly bronchial carcinoma, or from tracheal compression by lymphoma, Hodgkin's disease, etc.
5. Vascular causes as in pulmonary embolism or infarction, or in pulmonary oedema as a watery blood-tinged sputum, or rarely in pericarditis.
6. Tracheal compression from aneurysmal dilatation of the aorta gives the characteristic bovine cough, but this can also arise in left recurrent laryngeal nerve palsy.
7. Pneumoconiosis or collagen disorders affecting the lung.

*W hooping cough* is an acute respiratory infection with *Bordetella pertussis*, the characteristic paroxysmal stage of the disease being characterized by explosive bursts of sharp rapid coughs, followed by high-pitched whoops. Immunization of children has made the disease less common in Britain, but it can occur for the first time in adults.

## Sputum

Sputum production is always abnormal, the mucous glands of the respiratory tract producing 100 ml secretion in each 24 hours in health, but most of this is swallowed. *Purulent sputum* is usually yellow, a green colour suggesting that neutrophil peroxidase has been acting on the secretions for some time before expectoration. Not all purulent sputum is due to infection, as *sputum eosinophilia* may only be revealed by microscopic examination of purulent sputum. In pneumonia sputum is usually tough and sticky and may contain a small amount of blood as in the rusty spit of *Strep. pneunoniae* pneumonia. *Mucopurulent sputum* is characteristic of chronic bronchitis and emphysema, during an exacerbation. In bronchiectasis the patient usually coughs up a lot of sputum during the day and a change of position can often provoke further expectoration. *Serous or watery sputum* is characteristic of pulmonary oedema, and it is often blood-tinged.

## Haemoptysis

Haemoptysis is a major symptom of respiratory disease and every patient should always be asked the direct question 'Have you ever coughed up blood?'. If the patient says 'yes', four conditions must always be considered: bronchial carcinoma, tuberculosis, bronchiectasis and pulmonary infarction; but many other conditions can also cause haemoptysis. Blood-streaking of purulent spit is frequently found in pneumonia, lung abscess or bronchiectasis. Coughing-up of 'pure blood', that is without mucus or pus, is characteristic of tuberculosis, bronchiectasis or pulmonary infarction. Spots of blood in a mucoid sputum suggest bronchial carcinoma. Haemoptysis recurring repeatedly over several years probably indicates a benign lesion such as bronchiectasis, or very rarely idiopathic pulmonary haemosiderosis. Massive haemoptysis may occur in tuberculosis, lung abscess, bronchiectasis, bronchial carcinoma, and rarely mycetoma. Haemoptysis must always be investigated, with sputum smear for tuberculosis and chest radiograph, and if the cause is not then apparent, bronchoscopy and/or bronchography may be indicated. Despite full investigation, however, haemoptysis remains unexplained in up to 30–40% of cases, and repeated chest radiograph six weeks later, and possibly repeated bronchoscopy, may reveal a lesion which was not otherwise detectable. Haemoptysis can result from a lesion in the nose of pharynx and can be the presenting symptom of naso-pharyngeal carcinoma.

## Breathlessness

Breathlessness may be due to respiratory disease, cardiac disease or anaemia or of psychogenic origin. The pattern of breathlessness, its duration, associated symptoms and time course can all yield invaluable diagnostic information. Breathlessness is a symptom and not a sign, so that only the patient can say that he is breathless. It is an unpleasant sensation related to a feeling of increased demand for breathing. It should never be considered to arise from a psychogenic cause without positive evidence, coupled with absence of demonstrable organic disease. Breathlessness at rest is always abnormal, but clearly exer-tional breathlessness must be related to the severity of the exercise. Patients are more likely to be accurate in their recall of the number of flights of stairs they can climb before having to stop from breathless-ness, than in relating their breathlessness to the distance they can walk on the level, which is notoriously unreliable. It is diagnostically useful to consider the causes of breathlessness in relationship to the rate of onset of the symptoms, as below.

*Breathlessness developing suddenly* (at most an hour or so) may be due to:

1. An attack of bronchial asthma, when it is often associated with wheeze.

2. Pulmonary oedema, characteristically awaking the patient from sleep with cough and blood-tinged sputum.

3. Spontaneous pneumothorax, associated with chest pain, and breathlessness becoming progressively worse if a tension pneumo-thorax develops.

4. Pulmonary embolism, possibly with pleuritic pain of pulmonary infarction and haemoptysis, although these are often absent.

5. Pneumonia, again with pleuritic pain, sputum and haemoptysis, with fever being characteristic.

6. Rarer causes include laryngeal oedema, inhalation of a foreign body, the acute phase of allergic alveolitis, and exposure to an irritant gas.

*Breathlessness developing over weeks or months* is characteristic of:

1. Congestive heart failure (e.g. mitral stenosis, ischaemic heart disease, cor pulmonale, etc.).

2. Anaemia, when breathlessness on exertion usually means that the haemoglobin level is below 10 g/dl.

3. Pleural effusion of whatever aetiology, or diffuse fibrosing alveolitis of a subacute onset.

4. Breathlessness is common in late pregnancy, and in the obese.

5. Bronchial carcinoma can sometimes present with breathlessness due to occlusion of a major airway.

*Breathlessness progressing over months or years* may be due to:

1. Chronic bronchitis and emphysema.
2. Diffuse pulmonary fibrosis of whatever aetiology.
3. Pneumoconiosis.
4. Chronic pulmonary tuberculosis.
5. Thromboembolic or primary pulmonary hypertension.

## Wheeze

Wheeze is characteristic of airways obstruction, as for example in an attack of bronchial asthma, or in chronic bronchitis and emphysema. A dusty or smokey atmosphere may induce wheeze in the asthmatic, whereas the bronchitic will usually develop a cough in these circumstances. If asked, most asthmatics admit to being awakened from sleep with wheeze and breathlessness, from time to time. Tightness in the chest, when associated with wheeze, is more likely to be due to asthma (including exercise-induced asthma) than the angina of ischaemic heart disease, particularly if the symptom occurs in a young patient.

## Chest pain

Chest pain of respiratory origin is usually of two types:

1. Central chest pain, usually substernal and characteristically worse on coughing ('a red hot poker going down my throat'), as in tracheitis.
2. Pain felt laterally in the chest, with a stabbing quality, worse on breathing, and described as *pleuritic pain.*

Pleuritic pain can be mimicked by herpes zoster, which can be very confusing until the rash appears, or by other thoracic nerve lesions including vertebral collapse. However, it usually implies involvement of the pleura, as in pneumonia, pulmonary infarction, chest trauma (including fractured ribs), and rarely malignant disease. Shoulder tip pain can arise from irritation of either surface of the diaphragm, as pain referred from the C3 spinal segmental origin of the phrenic nerve. Mediastinal lesions, including bronchial carcinoma involving the hilar and paratracheal glands, can sometimes cause a dull central chest pain.

# Examination of the patient

Diagnostic clues may be obtained from general features, as well as the specific details of examination of the chest. Breathless patients often sit upright, and the patient with chronic bronchitis and emphysema characteristically has hunched-up shoulders, with apparent shorten-

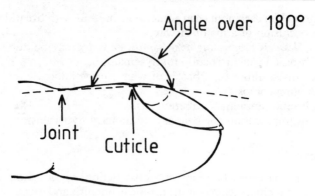

Angle over 180°

Joint   Cuticle

*Fig. 23.*    Clubbing of the fingers showing the increase in angle between the nail and nail bed

ing of his neck, the whole chest being held higher than normal. He may also purse his lips on expiration, and his breathlessness often causes him to talk in short sentences, which is also characteristic of the attack of acute bronchial asthma, if indeed the patient can speak at all. Characteristics of a cough may be obvious, but if not the patient should be asked to cough, when the presence of excess secretions in the airways will often be apparent by the moist sound. Hoarseness should always lead to enquiries as to the duration of the symptom. If for more than two or three weeks, a potentially serious cause should be suspected.

## The hands

The hands should be carefully examined for clubbing of the fingers, skin temperature and dilatation of forearm veins, muscle wasting and, of course, the radial pulses.

*Finger clubbing* is recognized by the loss of the angle between nail and nail bed (Fig. 23). It may be first seen in the index fingers; associated but less reliable signs include an increase in the volume of the terminal phalynx and curvature of the nail. The nail bed may be partially fluctuant, especially if the clubbing is of rapid onset, but minor degrees of fluctuation are very difficult to separate clearly from normal.

*Hypertrophic pulmonary osteoarthropathy* is an uncommon accompaniment of clubbing, with pain and swelling of wrists and ankles, with subperiostial new bone being demonstrable in the long bones on the radiograph. The blood flow to the fingers and toes is increased in clubbing. Clubbing is a recognized feature of:

1. Bronchial carcinoma.
2. Bronchiectasis.
3. Lung abscess and cystic fibrosis.
4. Fibrosing alveolitis and other forms of diffuse pulmonary fibrosis.
5. Empyema.
6. Long-standing pulmonary tuberculosis.
7. Mesothelioma and rarely other mediastinal tumour.
8. Subacute bacterial endocarditis.
9. Cyatonic congenital heart disease.
10. Primary bilary cirrhosis (rarely cirrhosis of other types).
11. Chronic diarrhoeal diseases including ulcerative colitis, Crohn's disease and malabsorption syndromes.

Clubbing also rarely occurs as a dominant hereditary form, when the patient's parents and/or siblings also have clubbing. By far the commonest cause of clubbing is bronchial carcinoma, and this should always be suspected in a patient in whom another cause is not obvious.

*An irregular flapping tremor*, best seen in the dorsiflexed out-stretched hands, is common in patients with acute carbon dioxide retention, but a similar sign can occur in patients with hepatic encephalopathy. However, carbon dioxide retention must be associated with hypoxia, and thus definite central cyanosis, if the patient is breathing air.

## Cyanosis

Central cyanosis is an important sign and requires recognition of an abnormal blue colour to the tongue. It is best recognized in daylight and may be more obvious by comparison with a colleague's tongue, if he is asked to place his head next to the patient's, and also put his tongue out, but only if he also does not have central cyanosis! All observers detect central cyanosis if the arterial oxygen saturation is below 85%, and most suspect its presence when the saturation is below 90%. It is recognized more readily in the polycythaemic than in the anaemic patient (see Chapter 9). Sulphhaemoglobinaemia and methaemoglobinaemia, the presence of rare abnormal blood pigments, also cause central cyanosis, but otherwise this sign always means arterial hypoxaemia. Peripheral cyanosis will always accompany central cyanosis, but differential cyanosis of the toes, but not the fingers, suggests persistent right-to-left flow through the patent ductus arteriosus.

## Stridor

Stridor is a musical sound best heard on inspiration, and results from narrowing of the glottis, trachea or major bronchi. It may be exaggerated by asking the patient to cough, followed by deep breathing with his mouth open. The narrowing may well result from external compression by tumour, or tumour within the airways.

## Inspection of the chest

An increased rate of breathing (or tachypnoea) must not be confused with the symptom of breathlessness. Tachypnoea of over 20–25/minute is typically found in pneumonia, pulmonary oedema, pulmonary infarction, diffuse pulmonary fibrosis, and anxiety — so that the rate should be counted unobtrusively. Accurate clinical assessment of the tidal volume is very difficult, and the alveolar ventilation is almost impossible to assess from merely watching the breathing. Marked continuous hyperventilation, however, where both rate and depth are increased so as to cause noisy breathing, is usually due to acidotic stimulation of the drive to breathing, as in renal acidosis or diabetic ketoacidosis, and is known as *Kussmaul's breathing*. Waxing and waning of the respiratory excursions, with a cycle length often of 30 seconds or more, characterizes *Cheyne-Stokes* respiration, which is usually an indication of cerebrovascular disease, but may arise rarely in left ventricular failure. Although the $P\text{CO}_2$ in these cases also waxes and wanes out of phase with respiration, Cheyne-Stokes respiration usually occurs on a background of central neurogenic hyperventilation. Marked depression of respiratory rate may be due to heroin or morphine overdosage, clinically confirmed by the small pupils.

*Bilateral indrawing of the intercostal spaces* is a reliable sign of *hyperinflation* of the chest, when it will be combined with indrawing of the supraclavicular fossae on inspiration. Localized unilateral indrawing may be a sign of localized bronchial obstruction with collapse of the underlying lobe. Indrawing is always pathological if seen over the pectoral regions, but may sometimes be seen in healthy thin subjects who are asked to take a deep breath, but only over the lower intercostal spaces. Hyperinflation is characteristic of chronic bronchitis and emphysema and during the acute attack of bronchial asthma. *Flattening* of the chest, just below the clavicles, suggest apical fibrosis. Paradoxical movement of the costal margins, whereby they move inwards during inspiration, may indicate diaphragmatic fatigue in a patient with severe chronic bronchitis and emphysema, in whom hyperinflation is present. An increase in the anteroposterior diameter of the chest (barrel-shaped chest), although widely regarded as indicating hyperinflation, can also arise from shortening of the thoracic spine (as in advancing age, vertebral collapse, etc.), and is therefore not a reliable sign of hyperinflation.

Kyphoscoliosis should always be noted, and position of the actual spinal processes located by palpation, as the kyphus or gibbus of the hunchback is usually formed by the angle of the ribs. Severe kyphoscoliosis can have serious effects on respiratory function.

## Palpation of the chest

*Diminished movement* of one side of the chest is always abnormal, indicating abnormal pathology on that side, but assessment of chest expansion is often badly performed. The sides of the chest should be symmetrically gripped with the fingertips, the thumbs lying very loosely on the skin, approximately at the midline or equidistant from it. Appreciation of asymmetrical movement is best made with the patient sitting on the side of a couch or bed, or sideways on a chair, with the examiner sitting centrally opposite to him. This position can be used to examine both the front and back of the chest when the patient turns round, and is usually far more comfortable for both patient and examiner.

The *apex beat* may be difficult to localize in patients with hyper-inflation due to chronic bronchitis and emphysema. Mediastinal shift can displace both the apex beat and the trachea, particularly in children, whereas in the adult usually only one is displaced, depending upon the site of the collapsed lobe.

*The position and mobility of the trachea* should be carefully noted. This can be done by the examiner's two thumbs being used to locate the trachea, after hooking them gently around both sternomastoids, then feeling the trachea between the thumbnails (Fig. 24). Slightly lowering the thumbs allows easy reference to the prominent medial ends of both clavicles, so allowing minor degrees of tracheal deviation to be readily appreciated. Gentleness and short thumbnails are essential! The length of the trachea outside the thorax can be estimated by the distance (in finger-breadths) between the cricoid cartilage (the signet ring cartilage lying below the thyroid cartilage) and the suprasternal notch (Fig. 25). Shortening of this distance to less than the usual three or four finger-breadths in the adult is a good sign of hyperinflation of the chest.

*Lymph gland enlargement* should be sought by careful palpation of the glands lying in the anterior and posterior triangles of the neck. Asking the patient to cough or give a forced expiration may move a node upwards so that it can be felt more easily by the palpating fingers. Particular attention is paid to the scalene nodes, which lie behind the clavicle, and the insertion of the scalene muscles into the first rib. These glands on each side may be palpated by an index finger, with the examiner standing behind the patient who has been asked to rotate his head downwards towards the side of examination. The examining finger then probes between the two heads of the sternomastoid. The axillary glands should also be examined, as, of course, should all other accessible lymph nodes as part of the general examination. It is

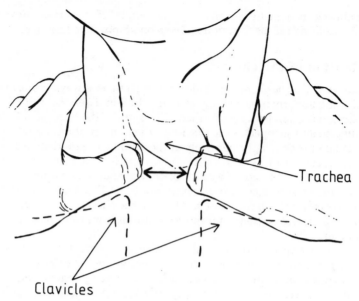

Clavicles

*Fig. 24.*    Locating the position of the trachea in relationship to the medial ends of both clavicles

convenient to palpate the female breast also whilst examining the chest, in search of nodules which may, of course, be malignant. Carcinoma of the breast can spread to the internal mammary nodes and is also a cause of malignant pleural effusion.

## Percussion of the chest

The finger to be percussed must be closely applied to the patient's skin without an intervening air space. A good (and elegant!) percussor uses only a flexion motion from the wrist, the percussed finger being struck vertically over the terminal phalyngeal joint by the percussing finger. Percussion notes include normal lung resonance, dullness and, rarely, hyper-resonance. Hyper-resonance (checked over one's own gastric gas bubble) is an unreliable sign of bilateral hyperinflation, for as with all physical signs comparison between the two sides is most valuable. Dullness of percussion is a reliable sign of pleural effusion, if combined with absence of breath sounds and diminished movement on the same side. Absence of the normal area of absolute cardiac dullness, behind the lower left quarter of the sternum (Fig. 26), is a valuable sign of chronic hyperflation of the chest. Loss of liver dullness is usually less certainly appreciated, but can also indicate hyperinflation. Tidal percussion of the bases of the lungs is really of

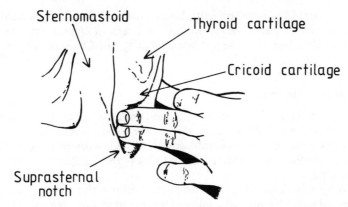

*Fig. 25.* Measuring the length of the trachea from the lower border of the cricoid cartilidge to the suprasternal notch, using finger-breadths. Shortening of this distance to below the normal three or finger-breadths is a good sign of hyperinflation of the chest

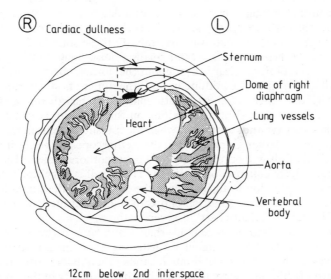

12cm below 2nd interspace

*Fig. 26.* Computerized axial tomogram of the chest, at 12 cm below the second intercostal space. The 'slice' is viewed from below upwards and shows the area of absolute cardiac dullness behind the lower left border of the sternum, in a normal subject, where lung (stippled area) does not intersopse between the chest wall and the heart

value only in a thin patient, but it may lead to a suspicion of diaphragmatic palsy, when the note appears to change little as the patient breathes. However, this is best confirmed by screening of the diaphragm radiologically.

## Auscultation of the chest

Use of the bell of the stethoscope is recommended, as the frequency and distribution of breath sounds, spoken sounds and most adventitious sounds are best transmitted by the bell, without the cut-off of lower frequencies which characterizes the diaphragm of the stethoscope.

*Noisy mouth breathing* can be heard without the stethoscope, but does not have the muscial quality of wheeze or stridor. Nevertheless, it correlates fairly well with severity of airways obstruction in patients with chronic bronchitis and emphysema or bronchial asthma. As with most breath sounds, this noise is produced by turbulence of air flow in the large air passages, where the linear velocity of flow is highest. The density of the respired gas can be reduced by breathing a mixture of 80% helium and 20% oxygen, so reducing this turbulence, and also the intensity of the breath sounds. The sounds heard at the chest wall are transmitted through air passages in adjoining lung, across the pleural space, through the chest wall, to the bell of the stethoscope. Disease anywhere along this pathway may modify these sounds.

*Vesicular breath sounds*, a faint rustling noise, longer in inspiration than expiration, are heard throughout the normal chest, apart from a small area near to the midline in both the upper chest anteriorly and posteriorly, where tracheal breath sounds are heard; this area may extend some 5 cm from the midline on the right upper chest of the adult. Breath sounds are absent when the transmission from the site of origin in the larger air passages to the stethoscope on the chest wall is impeded. This will occur locally, in a pneumothorax, pleural effusion or pulmonary collapse, or where the chest wall is very thick. Severe overall obstruction to air flow, as in the desperately ill asthmatic, may be associated with diminution of breath sounds throughout the chest, the dangerous 'silent chest' of severe asthma.

*Bronchial breathing* is harsher than vesicular breathing and has a hollow quality, best imitated by listening over one's own trachea. However, this latter sound is much harsher than that of true bronchial breathing, but does serve to remind one of the quality of the bronchial sounds. Inspiratory and expiratory phases of bronchial breathing are equal in duration and there is often a small gap between the inspiratory and expiratory sounds. Bronchial breathing is a reliable sign of consolidation of the underlying lung or lobes, but it can also be heard over pulmonary collapse and over the level of an effusion. Bronchial breathing over the lower lobes usually indicates that the bronchus supplying that region is patent, so allowing conduction of the sound generated from the trachea and larynx. Obstruction of this bronchus, causing absorption collapse behind the block, thus obliterates the bronchial breathing. In contrast, over the upper lobe, collapse may give rise to bronchial breathing, irrespective of whether the airway is open or closed, as the sound is transmitted from the trachea which is adjacent to the collapsed lobe, through the wall of the trachea, the collapsed lung, pleura and chest wall to the stethoscope.

*The spoken sounds* heard with the stethoscope (the traditional '99') are again conducted from the major airways to the chest wall. The high frequencies are transmitted most readily by consolidated lung, giving rise to *bronchophony*, when the actual number may be audible through the stethoscope. Bronchophony is characteristic of consolidation, but a better confirmatory sign is *whispering pectoriloquy*, when the sibilant sounds of the whisper are more readily transmitted through the consolidated lung to the stethoscope.

*Aegophony*, allegedly named after the goat-shaped Aegean sea, into which King Aegeus of Athens threw himself on being told of the black ails of his son Theseus's ship returning from the Minoan Court of Crete, reminded an earlier generation of physicians of a bleating goat. Today, one has to suffice by saying '99' when holding the nose, Aegophony can often indicate the upper level of a pleural effusion.

*Additional sounds* (rhonchi or wheezes) and crepitations (or crackles) and a pleural rub are not normally heard in health.

*Rhonchi*, or wheezes, indicate airways obstruction and may vary in pitch. Coarse rhonchi probably indicate obstruction in the larger air passages with secretions. However, it is not now considered that high-pitched rhonchi indicate obstruction in narrowed small airways, as it seems unlikely that the velocity of air flow, even in these narrowed airways, can generate such a high-pitched sound. Thus the sound is also thought to originate in the large air passages. A localized persistent rhonchus may occasionally arise from localized narrowing of a bronchus due to bronchial carcinoma or foreign body. High-pitched rhonchi are still a valuable sign in bronchial asthma, being clear objective measurements of airways obstruction, correlating reasonably with the $FEV_1$ or peak expiratory flow rate.

*Crepitations (or respiratory crackles)* are short discontinuous sounds varying in pitch and frequency. It now seems that these sounds arise from sudden opening of small airways which were previously closed, so that oscillation is produced in the walls of the small airways, so giving rise to the sound. The old attractive notion that they arose from bubbles breaking through a fluid in the airways, as when blowing down a straw into one's bottle of 'pop', no longer seems likely. Fine crepitations, occurring early in the inspiratory phase, are the hallmark of pulmonary oedema. Coarse crepitations, heard over a lobe or lobule, are suggestive of an inflammatory lesion, such as the first sign of an airspace pneumonia, but may also occur as the pneumonia resolves (redux crepitations). Bilateral basal crepitations occurring late in inspiration are characteristic of fibrosing alveolitis, or other types of diffuse pulmonary fibrosis. These crepitations may clear when the patient leans forward.

A *pleural rub*, likened to the creaking of a leather wallet, is a valuable sign of localized fibrinous pleurisy. The sound is present in both inspiration and expiration and is often associated with local pleural pain. The rub often vanishes as the pleural effusion develops, and thereby keeps the two inflamed surfaces apart. A rub may occasionally be confused with a coarse rhonchus (which clears on coughing), or a 'scapular creak', a sound which is exaggerated by movement of the scapula.

## Combinations of signs

Classical associations of signs from examination of the chest are:

1. *Pneumothorax*, with diminished movement, normal or hyper-resonant percussion note (very rarely dull), with absent breath sounds; mediastinal shift from the side of the lesion may be present in young patients with a tension pneumothorax.

2. *Pneumonic consolidation*, with diminished movement, dull percussion note and bronchial breathing with whispering pectoriloquy and/or bronchophony.

3. *Pleural effusion*, with diminished movement, dull or stony dull percussion note, absent breath sounds without mediastinal shift; rarely the mediastinum can shift from the side of the effusion, if this is very large, in a relatively young patient.

4. *Pulmonary collapse*, with diminished movement, dull percussion note, and mediastinal shift towards the side of the lesion, and possibly local indrawing of intercostal spaces, if the chest wall is thin.

5. *Diffuse pulmonary fibrosis and pulmonary oedema* both give rise to bilaterally reduced movement, usually with tachypnoea, and basal crepitations, early inspiration in pulmonary oedema, and late in inspiration in fibrosing alveolitis.

6. *Hyperinflation of the chest*, as in chronic bronchitis and emphysema, with bilateral indrawing of intercostal spaces, shortening of the cricosternal distance, absence of the normal cardiac dullness over the lower left quarter of the sternum, and increase of the subcostal angle.

## Further reading

COOPE, R. (1948) *Diseases of the Chest*, 2nd ed. Edinburgh: E. & S. Livingstone.
FORGACS, P. (1978) *Lung Sounds*. London: Baillière Tindall.

# 6

# Investigation of Respiratory Disease

The *chest radiograph* is essential for the accurate diagnosis and localization of diseases affecting thoracic anatomy, such as pneumonia, bronchial carcinoma, tuberculosis, pleural effusion, pneumothorax, etc., and may be equally important to exclude the presence of such diseases in patients with respiratory symptoms. However, the diagnosis and assessment of the severity of disease affecting the *function of the lungs*, as for example bronchial asthma, chronic bronchitis and emphysema, will also often require measurement of respiratory function. Determination of the cause of the disease, particularly if this is infective, will usually need *microbiological examination of sputum*, pleural effusions blood cultures, etc. Evidence that the body's immune systems are involved in a disease may be obtained by *skin prick test* (with an immediate reaction as indicating specific circulating IgE), the demonstration of circulating specific antibodies (precipitins in farmer's and bird-fancier's lung, or allergic aspergillosis), or delayed hypersensitivity (tuberculin skin test, etc.). Visualization of airways by fibreoptic or rigid *bronchoscopy* also allows biopsy of lesions, in both the bronchial wall and the lungs, so, for example, allowing proof of the cell type involved in a bronchial carcinoma, etc.

## The chest radiograph

The standard departmental film is a posteroanterior (PA) view, the X-ray tube being 2 m from the film, which is held against the front of the patient's chest. Bedside radiographs are usually anteroposterior (AP) views and may be taken with the patient supine; the X-ray tube is much closer to the patient, so magnifying structures near to the front of the chest, particularly the heart shadow. Films are normally taken at full inspiration (total lung capacity). The following technical factors should be assessed before an interpretation of the radiograph is attempted:

1. Is the film taken centrally, with the upper thoracic spine symmetrically placed between the medial ends of both clavicles? If

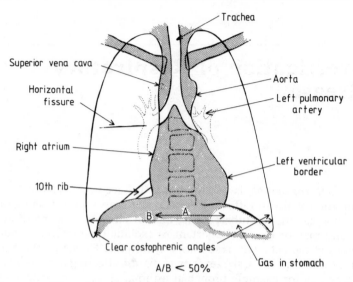

Trachea

Superior vena cava

Horizontal fissure

Right atrium

10th rib

Aorta

Left pulmonary artery

Left ventricular border

B ← A →

Clear costophrenic angles

A/B < 50%

Gas in stomach

*Fig. 27.*   Normal posteroanterior chest radiograph, in the central position, at full inspiration (tenth rib seen) and at correct exposure (vertebral outlines just seen through the heart shadow)

not, beware of interpreting the relative sizes of the hilar shadows, or of diagnosing mediastinal shift.

2. Has the patient taken a full inspiration? The upper borders of the diaphragms should be at least at the level of the tenth rib posteriorly. Films taken in relative expiration can increase the apparent heart diameter and make the lung fields appear plethoric.

3. Is the exposure correct? A faint outline of the vertebral bodies should just be discernible through the heart shadow in the PA film, down to at least three vertebral bodies above the diaphragm.

Look at the film on a viewing box, both close up and at a distance. Search the film systematically, starting with the body thorax, the ribs and pleura, the outer borders of the lung pattern, the diaphragm, and the heart borders. Then carefully compare the lung fields on each side, divided into the upper, mid and lower zones. The horizontal fissure should be identifiable on the posteroanterior view in 80% of normal cases, running from the centre of the right hilum to meet the sixth rib in the axilla. The oblique fissure is usually seen in the lateral view, ending on the diaphragm 2 cm or so behind its junction with the sternum. Abnormalities in position of the fissures must be explainable. The normal anatomical structures seen in the posteroanterior and lateral films are shown in Figs 27 and 28.

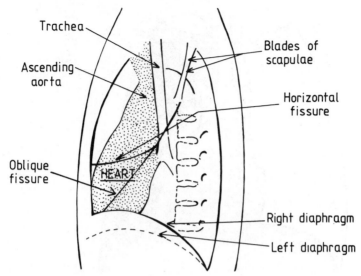

*Fig. 28.* The normal right lateral chest radiograph, showing some of the structures which should be identified

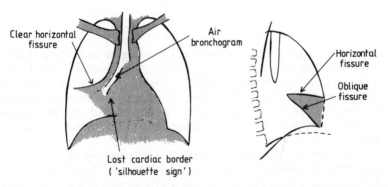

*Fig. 29.* Consolidation in the middle lobe, both posteroanterior and lateral view, showing the silhouette sign, with loss of cardiac border in the posteroanterior view

Characteristic radiographic patterns of disease include:

1. *Consolidation* (Fig. 29), which presents as a homogeneous or sometimes patchy opacity, usually based on the pleural or fissure interface, indicating lobar involvement. Loss of volume is not essential, but may be a characteristic of lobar consolidation behind an obstructed bronchus. Consolidation or collapse of a portion of the lung adjacent to the mediastinum or diaphragm obscures this border

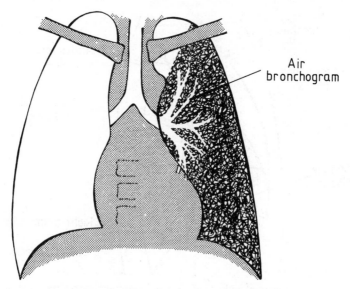

Air
bronchogram

*Fig. 30.*    Consolidation of the whole of the left lower lobe, showing a preserved 'air bronchogram' picture. Note that there is no loss of volume

('silhouette sign'). This is particularly valuable in differentiating middle lobe or lingular disease from the corresponding lower lobes. However, the lateral radiograph is essential to confirm these appearances and also to locate accurately the position of any radiographic abnormality in the lung fields. An *air bronchogram* may be seen within a consolidated lobe or segment if the supplying bronchus is patent (Fig. 30).

2. *Collapse* is radiologically identified as a homogeneous opacity with loss of volume. Collapse of the different lung lobes gives characteristic appearances (Fig. 31). Collapse of the left lower lobe may be missed entirely on the posteroanterior film and only revealed by a penetrated film, which shows the triangular opacity based on the vertebral column and diaphragm, behind the heart (Fig. 32). Loss of volume is shown by shift of the mediastinum towards the lesion, elevation of the hemidiaphragm, and occasionally crowding of ribs on the affected side.

3. *Pleural effusion* (Fig. 33) is recognized as a crescentia shadow higher on the lateral chest wall than medially, and obscuring the normal sharp costophrenic angle.

4. *Pneumothorax* is identified as a clear zone adjacent to the pleural surface, in which no lung markings are seen. The edge of the collapsed

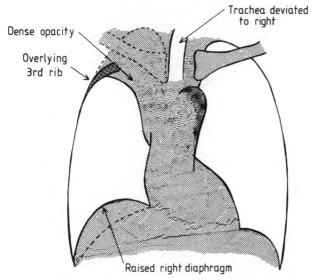

*Fig. 31.*   Collapse of right upper lobe, showing mediastinal shift in the trachea, elevation of the right diaphragm, and the homogenous dense opacity with marked upward coving of the transverse fissure, all indicating loss of volume in the collapsed lobe

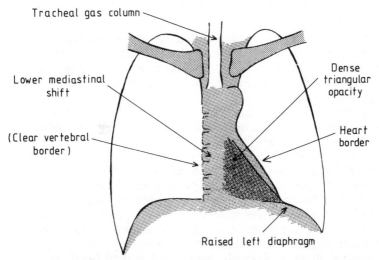

*Fig. 32.*   Collapse of the left lower lobe, showing as a dense triangular opacity behind the heart shadow in the posteroanterior film. Note the clear vertebral border, indicating the loss of volume and mediastinal shift to the left, and elevation of the left hemidiaphragm

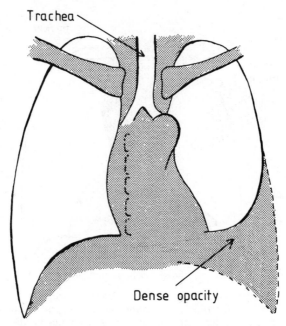

Trachea

Dense opacity

*Fig. 33.*     Left basal pleural effusion, showing the characteristic homogeneous opacity which rises higher in the lateral aspect of the
radiograph

lung may often be apparent, and an expiratory film may well
demonstrate a small pneumothorax which is not shown in the standard
film taken at full inspiration (total lung capacity). In tension pneumothorax the mediastinum may be shifted away from the
pneumothorax.

5. *Circumscribed lesions* ('coin lesions') (Fig. 34), with a clear
surrounding lung, may be difficult to detect if they lie over a rib and
may vary in diameter from a few millimetres to many centimetres.
Common causes of such discrete lesions include bronchial carcinoma
(uncalcified, diffuse outline with spicules, possibly ipsilateral hilar
gland enlargement, possibly diaphragmatic elevation); tuberculosis
(often calcified and most frequent in upper lobes, usually with satelite
lesions); haematogenous metastases (which may be multiple); rheumatoid nodules (peripheral, usually associated with overt rheumatoid
arthritis); hydatid cyst (common in endemic areas); and histoplasmosis
(common in endemic areas), usually with central calcification.

6. *Cavited lesions* suggest tuberculosis, squamous bronchial carcinoma (Fig. 35), lung abscess, rarely pulmonary infarction,
Wegener's granulomatosis, hydatid cyst or rheumatoid necrobiotic
nodules.

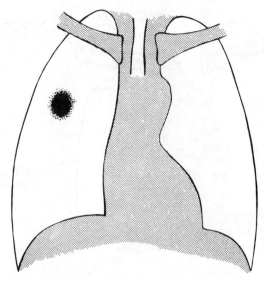

*Fig. 34.*    A typical coil lesion, which can occur anywhere in the lung fields; some possible causes are given in Table 1

*Table 1.    Causes of a coin lesion*

|  | Calcified | Cavitated |
|---|---|---|
| *Common* | | |
| Bronchial carcinoma | — | + |
| Solitary metastasis | — | (±) |
| Tuberculoma | + | (±) |
| Histoplasmoma } In endemic | + | — |
| Hydatid cyst } areas | — | + |
| *Rare* | | |
| Bronchial adenoma (particularly carcinoid) | — | — |
| Hamartoma ('chondroma') | + | — |
| Rheumatoid nodule | — | ± |
| Wegener's granulomatosis | — | ± |
| Arteriovenous fistula (30% telangiectasia) | (±) | — |
| Haematoma or infarct | — | ± |

7. *Diffuse infiltrates* of reticulonodular pattern may be due to coal-worker's pneumoconiosis (CWP), pulmonary oedema (with Kerley B lines, horizontal lines some 1 cm in length based on the lateral lung margin, best seen just above the costophrenic angles; also usually with

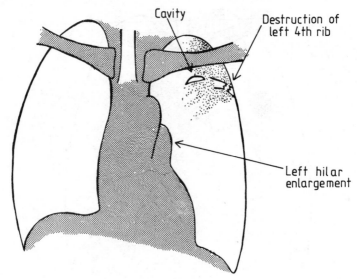

*Fig. 35.*    Cavitated squamous carcinoma of the left upper lobe, with left hilar gland enlargement, and local invasion with destruction of the left fourth rib

an enlarged heart) (Fig. 36), miliary tuberculosis, lymphangitis carcinomatosis, fibrosing alveolitis, allergic alveolitis, or sarcoidosis, the latter four usually being associated with loss of volume.

8. *Hilar adenopathy*, if unilateral, should always lead to suspicion of bronchial carcinoma with metastatic spread, but may also occur in pneumonia on the same side. If bilateral, sarcoidosis (stages I or II) or reticuloses are possibilities.

In many cases the most important method of diagnosing the cause of a radiographic abnormality is to *obtain a previous chest radiograph*. For example, a single circumscribed lesion which has not changed in size over one year is unlikely to be due to a bronchial carcinoma.

## Tomography

Standard radiographic technique is used to provide radiographic sections of the lungs at different levels by rotating the X-ray tube and the film about the patient during the exposure, so that only one part of the lung is clearly seen in focus. The technique is valuable to confirm the presence of cavitation, to assess the presence of calcium in a solid lesion, and also to characterize a mediastinal mass. Anteroposterior tomograms are usually numbered in centimetres from the table top, but the plane of the section should always be checked by referring to the rib structure which is most clearly seen in focus.

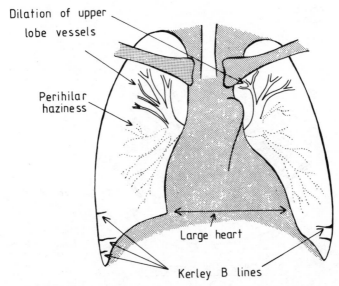

*Fig. 36.*    Pulmonary oedema with a large heart, dilatation of upper lobe vessels, perihilar haziness and Kerley B lines

## Barium swallow

Outlining the oesophagus with barium is useful in identifying mediastinal masses which may indent the oesophagus, for example in mediastinal gland enlargement from bronchial carcinoma. This may be an indication that a tumour is inoperable. *Diaphragmatic screening* may show paralysis of one hemidiaphragm, with upward movement of the affected side, when the patient is asked to sniff.

## CAT scans

Computerized axial tomography, a newly introduced and very expensive technique, which has already an established place in investigation of intracranial pathology, is being applied to the whole body (Fig. 37). In thoracic medicine the technique appears particularly valuable in estimating presence, size and characteristics of lesions of the mediastinum, pleura and possibly the lungs. Currently available machines cannot yield clear pictures of the heart; the scan time is too long. The technique produces transverse sections of the thorax, which are viewed from below upwards, and already appears valuable to detect presence and extent of mediastinal glandular enlargement, as in bronchial carcinoma (Fig. 38), and also can demonstrate metastatic deposits of tumour within the lungs which are not otherwise detectable by either conventional radiography or whole lung tomograms. Pleural

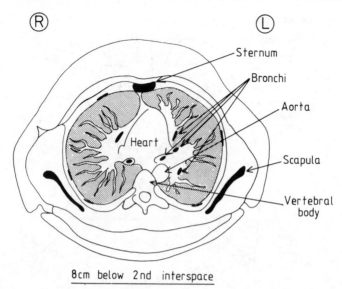

Ⓡ                                    Ⓛ

Sternum

Bronchi

Aorta

Heart

Scapula

Vertebral
body

8cm below 2nd interspace

*Fig. 37.*    Computerized axial tomogram of the chest, viewed from below,
the 'slice' being taken at 8 cm below the second intercostal space.
A compound picture showing the chest wall structures (vertebral
body, scapula, ribs and sternum, etc.), the mediastinal structures
(heart, aorta, etc.) and the branching bronchovascular markings
in the lung fields

lesions are clearly visualized, and the role of the technique in assessing
the extent and presence of emphysema, and also of diffusion interstitial fibrosis, is currently being evaluated. The current generation
of whole body scanners require that the patient should be capable of
holding his breath for at least 20 seconds, although the newer
generation of machines appear to be capable of producing adequate
scans with only a five second scan time or less.

# Respiratory function tests

*Simple spirometry*, with estimation of lung volumes by helium
dilution, combined with measurements of $FEV_1$ and FVC, will allow
characterization of obstructive or restrictive patterns (see Chapter 1).
*Arterial blood gas analysis* will confirm the presence of arterial
hypoxaemia, which may be suspected from central cyanosis, and also
define the type of any respiratory failure (see Chapter 11), and of an
acid–base disturbance (see Chapter 3). Measurement of transfer factor
for carbon monoxide ($TCO$), in combination with the above studies,
may allow characterization of a restrictive pattern, or suggest that a

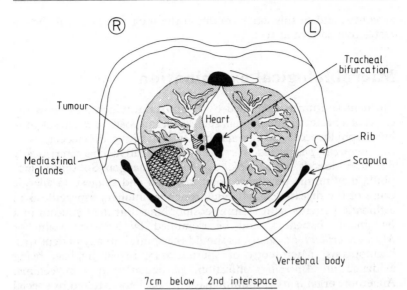

Ⓡ                                    Ⓛ

Tracheal bifurcation

Tumour

Heart

Rib

Mediastinal glands

Scapula

Vertebral body

7cm below 2nd interspace

*Fig. 38.*     Computerized axial tomogram of the chest, viewed from below, the 'slice' being taken at 7 cm below the second intercostal space. A peripheral bronchial carcinoma with spread to mediastinal glands shown in the right lung, again being a composite view showing mediastinal and chest wall structures, along with the structures within the lungs (stippled areas)

patient with an obstructive pattern has also a considerable degree of emphysema if the $T$CO is particularly low for the level of airways obstruction and hyperinflation. Variability of airways obstruction, either spontaneously or in response to treatment, is the characteristic feature of bronchial asthma. Measurement of $FEV_1$ or peak flow following exercise, or after inhalation of a suspected allergen (bronchial provocation test), can sometimes be used to prove that a specific allergen is causing the asthmatic attack. Similar measurements may be used to work to characterize occupational asthma (see Chapter 17).

*Exercise testing,* whereby measurements of minute ventilation, tidal volume, heart rate, and arterial oxygen saturation from non-invasive ear oximetry, are related to the severity of exercise as assessed by the oxygen uptake, can be very useful to define the cause of a complaint of breathlessness on exertion, if this is not apparent from the history, clinical examination, chest radiography, etc. In recurrent pulmonary thromboembolism clinical examination and chest radiograph may be normal, and hyperventilation and arterial desaturation are characteristic findings during progressive exercise. This is also seen in fibrosing alveolitis, and in this latter condition the lung volumes will show a restrictive pattern at rest.

# Microbiological examination

Purulent sputum is examined by Gram stain, which may show the cause of a bacterial pneumonia, such as Gram-positive cocci, suggesting staphylococcal pneumonia; or Gram-positive diplococci, as in *Streptococcus pneumoniae*; or the Gram-negative characteristically pleomorphic rods of *Haemophilus influenzae* infection. Sputum eosinophilia may mimic purulence from infection and suggest an allergic cause of the disease, e.g. allergic bronchopulmonary aspergillosis in asthmatic patients with sputum eosinophilia. Purulent sputum in a pneumonic patient should be examined by acid-fast stain for *Mycobacterium tuberculosis*, as should the sputum in any patient with haemoptysis. Microscopy of sputum may reveal hyphae, being evidence of *Aspergillus* infection, particularly in a mycetoma. Anaerobic organisms in sputum may only be demonstrated by special culture techniques, but as anaerobes are commonly found in the mouth, care must be taken that such specimens are obtained from the lower respiratory tract.

Viral infections may be shown by growth of the virus from nasal washings, using special transport medium to convey the washings to the laboratory. A four-fold rise in the antibody titre in paired sera taken over a 10-day interval is the usual method of proving a viral nature of a respiratory infection.

Blood cultures should be considered in any febrile patient, particularly if the response to apparently appropriate antibiotics is delayed for more than 48 hours.

# Bronchoscopy

Direct inspection of the bronchial tree is a major means of diagnosing bronchial carcinoma and should be considered in every patient in whom haemoptysis is not established to arise from another cause, or in those patients in whom pneumonia shows no resolution over a period of one or two weeks. The rigid bronchoscope requires extensive local or even general anaesthesia, and a patient whose neck can be hyper-extended. Most bronchoscopic examinations today are carried out by the flexible fibreoptic instrument (Fig. 39), passed directly through the nose, under local anaesthesia (lignocaine 40 mg/litre, total dose not exceeding 5 ml) with premedication by papaveretum 20 mg and hyoscine hydrobromide 0.4 mg (Omnopon-Scopolamine) intramuscularly one hour previously. The dose of premedication is reduced in

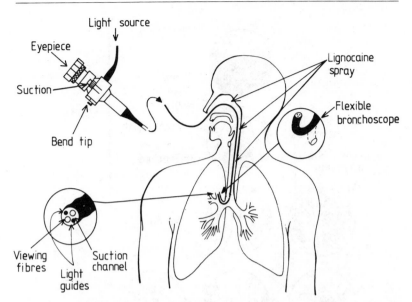

*Fig. 39.*   Fibreoptic bronchoscopy, showing the instrument passed through the nose under local anaesthesia, in the seated or supine patient. The flexible instrument contains light guides and a narrow suction channel through which the special biopsy forceps, wire brushes, flexible suction biopsy needle, or bacterial sampling catheter can all be passed. The tip is steerable, through the angles shown in the inset

patients with known carbon dioxide retention. The flexible fibrescope allows inspection of the orifices of all 19 lobar bronchi, and often beyond (Figs 2, 40). Lesions seen can be biopsied directly with cutting forceps passed through the fibreoptic bronchoscope, but diagnostic material can also be obtained from brushings or washings of suspicious lesions. The new technique of transbronchial suction needle biopsy, through the fibreoptic bronchoscope, can also provide a histological diagnosis in many cases, even if the lesion itself is not clearly visible. Transbronchial biopsy of lung tissue through the fibrescope is now known to be a safe procedure which may yield diagnostic tissue, particularly in sarcoidosis, and less frequently in diffuse interstitial lung disease.

The rigid bronchoscope is preferred to the fibreoptic bronchoscope for removal of foreign bodies from the bronchial tree, control of massive haemoptysis, and lavage of copious, viscid bronchial secretions. Minor hypoxaemia during fibreoptic bronchoscopy is readily corrected by oxygen given through the other nostril. Bronchoalveolar lavage, using repeated aliquots of saline instilled and then aspirated from a lobar segmental bronchus, can yield cells from deep within the

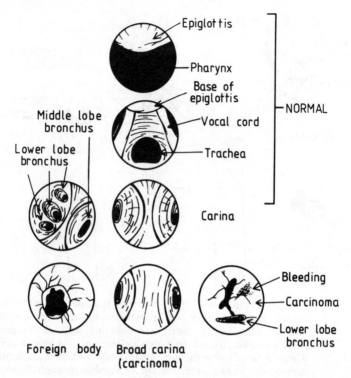

*Fig. 40.*    Appearances seen through the fibreoptic bronchoscope. The
instrument is passed through the nose, showing first the epi-
glottis, then the vocal chords, the main carina, then appearances
in a lower lobe bronchus and the origin of the middle lobe
bronchus. Examples of pathological lesions are shown below; a
foreign body in a lobar bronchus; widening of the main carina by
carcinomatous glands; and the appearances of bronchial carcinoma with some bleeding

lungs. These cells include lymphocytes, pulmonary alveolar macrophages (PAM), polymorphonuclear leucocytes (PMN) and eosinophils. A differential cell count on these lavage fluids may thus yield
important diagnostic information, particularly in interstitial lung
disease, but this subject is rapidly developing as experinece
accumulates.

## Further reading

GEE, J. B. and Fick, R. B. (1980) Bronchoalveolar lavage. *Thorax*, **35**, 1–8.
ISHERWOOD, I. and BEST, J. J. K. (1980) Uses of computed tomography in lung
    disease. In *Recent Advances in Respiratory Medicine II*, ed. D. C. Flenley.
    Edinburgh: Churchill Livingstone.

MINTZNER, R. A., MALAVE, S. R., NIEMAN, H. L. et al. (1979) Computer vs. conventional tomography in evaluation of primary and secondary pulmonary neoplasms. *Radiology*, **132**, 653–659.

MITCHELL, D. M. and COLLINS, J. V. (1980) Fibreoptic bronchoscopy. In *Recent Advances in Respiratory Medicine II*, ed. D. C. Flenley. Edinburgh: Churchill Livingstone.

SIMON, G. (1978) *Principles of Chest X-ray Diagnosis*, 4th ed. London: Butterworths.

SPENCER, H. (1977) *Pathology of the Lung*, 3rd ed., vols 1 and 2. Philadelphia: W. B. Saunders.

STRADLING, P. (1976) *Diagnostic Bronchoscopy*, 3rd ed. Edinburgh: Churchill Livingstone.

# 7

# Acute Upper Respiratory Tract Infections

Upper respiratory tract infections account for half of the total time lost from work in Britain. On average a person has five such episodes in a year, but usually only sees his doctor for one of these. These conditions tend to fall into three patterns, coryza, acute sore throat and influenza.

## The coryza syndrome (common cold)

This well known, self-limiting syndrome is caused by viral infection and is spread by person-to-person contact. Sneezing, headache, malaise and chills are prominent, with nasal discharge and sore throat. Fever is rare, and these constitutional symptoms last for only one or two days. Initially the nasal discharge is clear, watery and profuse, but later becomes mucopurulent and more tenacious. Recognized causal agents of the coryza syndrome include parainfluenza viruses, coronavirus, Coxsackie viruses (particularly A21 and A24) and the rhinoviruses. Children under four are particularly prone to coryza, when the infection is spread to them by school contacts from older children. People over 40 tend to suffer less frequent colds, but, of course, the syndrome is commoner in winter and autumn. Secondary bacterial infection is rarely significant, although *H. influenzae* and *Strep. pneumoniae* can often be grown from the purulent nasal secretions, but these may well be normal commensals in the nose. Treatment with antibiotics is therefore not justifiable for the common cold, unless the rare complications such as sinusitis, otitis media, acute bacterial bronchitis, or pneumonia develop. Aspirin, hot drinks, and possibly bed rest for a day or two give the traditional (and often necessary) symptomatic relief.

## Acute sore throat

This is the commonest respiratory symptom which brings patients to their doctor, and although some 80% of cases may be viral in origin, other possibilities should always be considered. The causes may be:

1. *Acute pharyngitis of viral origin*, of which the dominant symptom is sore throat, is usually associated with fever and headache, the pharynx being inflammed, with enlarged tonsils and adenoids, with patchy yellow exudate on the tonsils and tender maxillary lymph nodes. Adenoviruses or Coxsackie viruses are the usual culprits, and the condition may occur in epidemics, particularly among military recruits and other closed communities. However, sporadic cases are very common in other populations.

2. *Streptococcal sore throat* is often clinically indistinguishable from viral pharyngitis, but fever is usually more pronounced, and there is usually little cough. A throat swab yielding group A streptococci is not diagnostic of this condition, for this may be a normal throat commensal. Nonetheless, most doctors give penicillin or erythromycin if this organism is found, for although this will have little effect on the acute syndrome, it will prevent *rheumatic fever*. However, it is not certain that such antibiotic treatment will prevent post-streptococcal acute nephritis. Ampicillin or amoxycillin should *not* be prescribed for sore throat, as this may be due to infectious mononucleosis, where these antibiotics usually produce a skin reaction of varying severity.

3. *Infectious mononucleosis* (IM), an acute self-limited disease of young adults, often starts as fever with sore throat, lymphadenopathy, and usually splenomegaly. Most cases are caused by Epstein-Barr virus (EBV), which may be transmitted by kissing, with an incubation period of 30–50 days. EB virus infection in early life causes few symptoms, infectious mononucleosis then being rare. If, however, EB infection is delayed until young adult life, infectious mononucleosis is a common consequence. High and lasting immunity follows EBV infections.

Infectious mononucleosis starts abruptly, with fatigue, sweating and chills, followed by headaches which last for three or four days, with photophobia. Fever usually lasts for a few days, and rarely for as long as three weeks. Some 85% of patients have sore throat, lasting for about a week. The larynx may be inflamed, but is rarely ulcerated, the appearances being similar to haemolytic streptococcal infection. Petechial haemorrhages confined to the soft palate are said to be diagnostic of infectious mononucleosis. Lymphadenopathy characteristically involves the posterior cervical nodes, but all groups of lymph nodes in the body may be involved. Splenomegaly occurs in over half the patients, and hepatomegaly probably in a quarter. The blood count reveals lymphocytosis with atypical mononuclear cells. A heterophil IgM is shown by the Paul-Bunnell test. If this IgM is partially absorbed by guinea-pig serum, the result is diagnostic of infectious mononucleosis and this test will be positive in 90% of patients within the first three weeks. The Monospot test is a useful screening method. Ampicillin, often erroneously given under supposition that the patient is suffering from a streptococcal or other bacterial sore throat, produces a skin rash in over 80% of patients. However, permanent ampicillin sensitivity does not develop.

4. *Herpangina*, usually due to Coxsackie virus or, rarely, echovirus infection in infants and young children, presents as headache with anorexia, vomiting and abdominal pain, with fever and sore throat. The pharynx shows papulovesicular or ulcerated lesions with marked erythema on the tonsils, and this may spread on to the anterior pillars of the fauces, the soft palate and uvula. The condition usually lasts four to six days.

5. *Diphtheria* is rare in developed countries, for immunization programmes have almost eliminated the disease from residents of these countries, so that even the unimmunized have little chance of contracting the infection. The incubation period is one to seven days, after which few constitutional symptoms develop, with low-grade fever. Local pain in the throat is then associated with a soft exudate on the tonsils and pharynx. This initial exudate wipes off easily, but later extends to become thick and grey, and then bleeds when removal is attempted. Laryngeal diphtheria can cause respiratory obstruction, myocarditis (with ventricular arrhythmias) and cranial nerve palsies, which latter arise typically two to six weeks after the onset. Visual accommodation problems and nasal regurgitation due to palatal palsy are characteristic. Isolation, bed rest and antitoxins are mandatory for treatment. Antibiotics do not affect the course of the disease, but prevent the development of a carrier stage.

6. *Acute leukaemia or agranulocytosis* may present as sore throat due to lack of antibacterial defences from B and T lymphocytes, and/or polymorphonuclear leucocytes. Anaemia, possibly purpura and other signs of infection give a clue to the diagnosis, which is, of course, confirmed by examination of the peripheral blood and bone marrow.

# Influenza

Influenza is an acute contagious disease occurring in localized outbreaks, epidemics, and rarely pandemics throughout the world. The influenza virus is an RNA virus with three antigenic types, which are distinguished by haemagglutinin (H) and neuraminidase (N) antigens, which are carried in the outer coat. Type A virus causes pandemics and local epidemics, whereas B strains cause localized outbreaks and sporadic cases. Type A virus undergoes antigenic shift, whereby a change in the H and A antigens occurs spontaneously. This can thus lead to pandemics, as many potential hosts have no antibodies to these new strains of A virus. Pandemics occurred in 1889–92, 1918–19 (which killed more people throughout the world than did the Great War of 1914–18) and most recently in 1957–8 (Asia 57 strain). Outbreaks usually start abruptly, with up to half the population being rapidly affected, the peak incidence usually occurring within three weeks from start of the epidemic. A whole epidemic may be over within six weeks, but, of course, air travel allows new strains of virus to spread throughout the world very rapidly.

After an incubation period of one to three days, the illness starts with an abrupt onset of fever, sweating and headache, with muscular aches and pains. A non-productive painful cough is usual, often associated with conjunctival irritation and nasal obstruction. Bronchitis and croup are common in children, but usually resolve within a few days if there are no complications. The main danger of influenza lies in the complication of staphylococcal pneumonia. Before the antibiotic era this was extremely lethal, and still carries a high mortality. Pneumonia from *Strep. pneumoniae* and *H. influenzae* secondary infection is also well recognized, and patients with chronic bronchitis and emphysema, or mitral stenosis and congested lungs are particularly prone to these complications. The virus can be isolated from nasal washings, but the diagnosis can also be proved by a rise in antibody titres. Complicating pneumonia of bacterial origin is confirmed by Gram stain of the sputum. Specific antibiotic therapy is mandatory for such secondary infections, but, of course, has no effect on the underlying influenza.

*Prophylaxis*, using killed *vaccine*, is now recommended for patients who are prone to influenza, such as those with chronic bronchitis and emphysema, other chronic respiratory diseases, and valvular heart disease. Unfortunately, a specific vaccine cannot be prepared in time to protect against a sudden antigenic shift in influenza A, which usually leads to influenza epidemics, if not pandemics. Vaccination is given by intramuscular injection each autumn, using the strains recommended as being likely to be prevalent in the forthcoming winter. Immunization is not usually associated with any systemic disturbance. Occasionally a sore arm and a mild fever may occur.

# Acute tracheitis and bronchitis

Many of the above viral syndromes of the upper respiratory tract may be complicated by tracheitis and bronchitis, and these may also complicate measles and whooping cough, particularly in children. Bronchitis is indicated by an irritating dry cough with retrosternal soreness, like a 'red hot poker going down my throat'. Cigarettes and other atmospheric pollutants provoke the cough and even hardened smokers nearly always stop smoking at least while they have acute tracheitis. Wheeze and breathlessness suggest spread of infection to bronchi, and the cough may then be productive of mucopurulent sputum. 'Recurrent acute bronchitis' is a dangerous diagnosis to make and should always raise the possibility of underlying tuberculosis, chronic bronchitis and emphysema, or bronchial carcinoma as the cause of a persistent or recurrent cough with or without sputum.

Antibiotic treatment of acute bronchitis or tracheitis is indicated when the sputum becomes purulent, as *Strep. pneumoniae* and *H. influenzae* are then commonly found to be present. Ampicillin 500 mg four times daily for a 10-day course is appropriate. Suppression of cough is important, as this may be painful and keep the patient awake. Codeine phosphate in adequate dosage (15–30 mg) by mouth can suppress cough, but also carries a definite risk of respiratory depression in a patient with chronic bronchitis and emphysema, particularly if he has pre-existing type II respiratory failure with hypoxia and an elevated $PCO_2$ (Chapter 11). Pholcodine (10 mg) is as effective as 15 mg of morphine in suppressing the cough, but strong narcotics, such as morphine and methadone, although effective cough suppressants, should clearly be avoided in treating such a benign condition. Wheeze associated with a cough can often be relieved by terbutaline or salbutamol in a metered dose aerosol, possibly combined with ipratropium bromide in the older patient. Steam inhalations are an effective symptomatic remedy for viscid secretions and can be provided by a boiling electric kettle near the patient, but beware of burns!

## Further reading

KILBOURNE, E. D. (1975) *The Influenze Viruses and Influenza.* New York: Academic Press.

KNIGHT, V. (1973) *Viral and Mycoplasmal Infections of the Respiratory Tract.* Philadelphia; Lea and Febiger.

SHURIN, S. B. (1979) Infectious mononucleosis. *Pediat. Clins N. Am.,* **26**, 315–326.

STUART-HARRIS, C. (1979) Epidemiology of influenza in man. *Br. med. Bull.,* **35**, 3–8.

YOSHIKAWA, T. T., CHOW, A. W. and GUZE, L. B. (1980) *Infectious Diseases: Diagnosis and Management.* Boston: Houghton Mifflin.

# 8

# Pneumonia

Pneumonia has been used to describe the illness resulting from lung inflammation since the days of Hippocrates, and remains the recommended term when the inflammation results from infection. The 'upstart' term pneumonitis seems best reserved for lung inflammation resulting from chemical or physical injury, as in the chemical pneumonitis following inhalation of acid, or in radiation pneumonitis to describe the acute lung reaction to ionizing radiation. The need to preserve sterility in the lung parenchyma, where conditions are otherwise ideal for microbial growth, has led to the evolution of a formidable array of lung defences against infection (see Chapter 2). Failure of these mechanisms predisposes to pneumonia, which can be simply described as virulence of the invading organisms exceeding the capacity of the host defences. Thus in previously healthy subjects living in the community, only very virulent strains of the *Streptococcus pneumoniae* (Types 1, 3, 4, 7, 8 and 12) can commonly cause pneumonia; whereas hospital-acquired pneumonia in patients with suppression of their immune system is often due to organisms of low virulence, such as *Pneumocystis carinii*, invasive aspergillosis etc.

## Epidemiology

The early triumphs of the sulphonamides and antibiotics were well shown in the declining death rates from pneumonia. Thirty to 40 years ago this was particularly apparent in young adults, but this has not continued in the deaths from pneumonia in patients over 70, where there has been very little change in recent years (Fig. 41). Closed communities are particularly susceptible to pneumonia, for example in army recruits, black gold-miners in South Africa, and the highlanders of Papua New Guinea who live in communal long houses. Similar close contacts, presumably leading to person-to-person spread by droplets, may account for the intermittent mini-epidemics of pneumonia which occur from time to time in geriatric hospitals.

## Classification

The simple ideal of classifying pneumonia by the infective agent is unfortunately often impossible, as this may never be found.

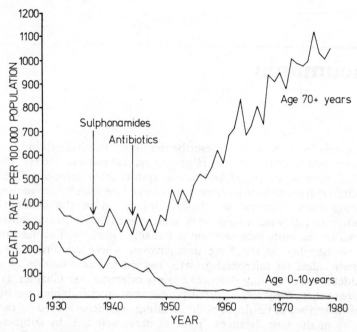

*Fig. 41.*    Death rates from pneumonia in men, 1931–79, in England and
Wales, for those aged 0–10 years, showing a marked fall. A similar
fall has not occurred, despite sulphonamides and antibiotics, in
those over 70 years

Furthermore, the presenting clinical features of pneumonia are often
very similar despite different causal organisms, and some cases of
pneumonia may be due to multiple agents, as in aspiration pneumonia,
or when staphylococcal pneumonia complicates influenza. Pneumonia
*acquired in the community* is usually due to *Streprococcus pneumoniae*, a
virus or *Mycoplasma pneumoniae*, whereas *hospital-acquired pneumonia*, often much more serious than that acquired in the community,
may be due to *Pseudomonas, Klebsiella* or other Gram-negative
organisms, sometimes with fungal super-infection, or anaerobic
infection. Pneumonia in these circumstances is usually a complication
in patients with impaired cellular or humoral immunity, or defective
polymorphonuclear phagocytosis, or from impairment of mechanical
defences of the respiratory tract, notably the cough reflex.

   The most practical clinical classification depends upon the radiographic appearances, this being substantiated by an aetiological diagnosis if and when the causative organism is isolated.

*Lobar pneumonia*, involving the air spaces within an anatomically recognized lobe of the lung (although the whole lobe is rarely involved, at least initially), is also known as air space or alveolar pneumonia. It implies pneumonic consolidation in the alveoli, usually sparing the major bronchi, so giving rise to the characteristic radiographic appearance of an *air bronchogram* (see Fig. 30), where the patent major air-containing bronchi are outlined by the surrounding consolidated alveoli. This pattern is most commonly seen in pneumonia due to *Streptococcus pneumoniae*, but early treatment with penicillin usually prevents full development of the lobar consolidation.

*Bronchopneumonia*, where the inflammatory process starts in the conducting airways and spreads to the surrounding alveoli, if often patchy and bilateral, and may arise from a mixed infection with *Strep. pneumoniae* and *Haemophilus influenzae*, as in an exacerbation of chronic bronchitis and emphysema, but bronchopneumonia can also occur in staphylococcal pneumonia.

*Interstitial pneumonia*, initially presenting as a fine reticular pattern, usually bilaterally, although asymmetrical, and then progressing to air space consolidation, is often the characteristic radiographical appearance of a pneumonia due to *Mycoplasma*, rickettsiae, or virus infection.

# Pneumococcal pneumonia (Strep. pneumoniae)

This is the commonest bacterial pneumonia, affecting all age groups, but with the highest incidence in the old. Alcoholics, cirrhotics, diabetics and patients with renal failure, multiple myeloma, leukaemia or lymphoma are all at greater risk of developing pneumococcal pneumonia, as are those with sickle cell anaemia or who have had a splenectomy.

*Streptococcus pneumoniae* are lanceolate paired organisms, which can appear in short chains, and are identified as *Gram-positive* organisms in stained specimens of sputum. Virulent organisms are encapsulated, the type-specific polysaccharide antigen being found in the capsule. Eighty-two serotypes are known, but types 8, 4, 5, 12, 3, 1, 7 and 9 (in declining order of frequency) cause most human infections, type 3 being a particularly virulent organism. Pneumococcal antigen can be detected by countercurrent immunoelectrophoresis (CIE) in the serum in over 50% of patients with pneumococcal lobar pneumonia, and can thus be a valuable diagnostic aid. A vaccine containing 14 of the most common antigen types is now available, but its value in preventing pneumococcal pneumonia in patients with chronic bronchitis and emphysema, or those following splenectomy, or in chronic cardiac or renal disease is currently being evaluated.

## Pathogenesis

*Streptococcus pneumoniae*, inhaled into the trachea, usually lands on the mucociliary blanket in small airways, or in alveoli in the lower or middle lobes. In the immune individual the polysaccharide capsular antigen of the pneumococcus binds to anti-pneumococcal secretory IgA in the mucociliary blanket, with resultant release of vasoactive peptides from adjacent mast cells (histamine, kinins etc.) which join with ill-defined bacterial toxins to initiate an intense inflammatory response within the alveoli. This is characterized by vasodilatation and disruption of the tight junctions of Type I alveolar epithelial cells, so allowing plasma exudate to flood into the alveoli. The pneumococci rapidly multiply in this fluid, and so sweep through an affected lobe, passing from alveolus to alveolus through the pores of Kohn, to the pleural surface, to end by exciting the fibrinous pleurisy which causes the characteristic pleuritic pain. In the non-immune individual the intense inflammation leads within a few days to the secretion of IgM antibody (the earliest immune response to the infection) in the alveolar exudate, in spite of its large size of 900 000 daltons, as it passes through the disrupted alveolar epithelium. Specific IgM, and later specific IgG and IgA, antibodies are synthesized from plasma cell transformation of B lymphocytes, following the binding of the polysaccharide antigen to specific immunoglobulin surface receptors on the B lymphocyte. The pneumococci are carried to the local lymph nodes and also to bronchus-associated lymphoid tissue (BALT) by the rich pulmonary lymphatic bed, and there meet both macrophages and B and T lymphocytes.

Antigen binding to specific IgM (and later IgG) activates the complement system, components of which are present in the alveolar exudate, by the classical pathway, with C3b amplification using the alternative pathway after primary cleavage of the C3 component. Other products of this critical C3 cleavage (C3a and d) and later complement components (C5a etc.) act as anaphylotoxins to release further vasoactive peptides from mast cells, and also chemotactically attract polymorphonuclear leucocytes. These diapedese in increasing numbers into the alveolar exudate through the capillaries, being in turn replaced from the great potential store of these cells in the bone marrow, as shown by the characteristic polymorphonuclear leuco-cytosis in the blood of the patient with lobar pneumonia.

These polymorphonuclear leucocytes are the major killers of pneumococci within the first 24–48 hours of the illness, and many of the cells die in this endeavour. The bacteria, opsonized by surface binding of specific IgA before being phagocytosed, are killed intracellularly by subsequent fusion of the intracellular lysosomes with the phagosome, so releasing the myeloperoxidase–hydrogen peroxide–halide bacterial killer enzymes into the phagosomes. The latter addition of singlet oxygen ($O^-$) within the cell completes the bacterial killing, but often also results in death of the polymorphonuclear leucocyte. This cell is unique amongst body cells in containing no superoxide dismutase to protect against singlet oxygen.

Alveolar macrophages, and other monocytes recruited from the blood stream, then in turn ingest many of the dead polymorphonuclear leucocytes, stimulated by lymphokines released from T lymphocytes, as part of the cellular immune response to the infection. Resolution is finally complete, with digestion of the fibrinous exudate by enzymes from the dying polymorphonuclear leucocytes and restoration of normal alveolar architecture from metaplasia of Type II alveolar cells to replenish any deficiency of Type I epithelial surface cells. Surfactant is then once again resynthesized, so allowing the alveolus to become air-filled, and so participate in respiratory gas exchange.

## Clinical features

In healthy adults the illness is often acute in onset, with shivers or rigor and the temperature rising rapidly to 38–39°C. Pleuritic pain, usually laterally in the lower chest, or in the shoulder tip in diaphragmatic pleurisy, is characteristic. The developing cough aggravates the pain and may make the raising of the viscid blood-stained rusty sputum very distressing. The patient is breathless and ill.

The earliest signs in the chest are diminished movement of the affected side, with reduced breath sounds, followed by fine crepitations with dullness to percussion, which precedes the development of full-blown consolidation with bronchial breathing and whispering pectoriloquy. A pleural rub may be heard over the site of maximum pleuritic pain, but the rub vanishes as a small pleural effusion develops. Resolution is indicated clinically by the redux coarse crepitations which last for a few days. Central cyanosis indicates hypoxaemia, the arterial oxygen saturation then being below 90%, and this can be confirmed by arterial blood gas analysis, which will show the characteristic picture of hypoxaemia with a low $PCO_2$ and respiratory alkalosis. Labial herpes occurs in some 10% of cases, from the fever reactivating the latent HSV-1 virus infection which is probably present in 90% of all adults. Polymorphonuclear leucocytosis, with the white count reaching 20 000–30 000 is characteristic, and in severe cases. *Strep. pneumoniae* may be recovered from blood culture. *Empyema*, classically heralded by a later secondary rise in temperature, can be confirmed by aspiration of purulent pleural fluid, but this is very uncommon in patients who are treated with antibiotics. The other complications are bacteraemia, including meningitis, endocarditis and peritonitis, but are also very rare in the antibiotic era.

# Radiology

An homogeneous or patchy opacity abutting against a pleural surface is characteristic, the air bronchogram (if present) indicating that the major airways are patent (see Fig. 30). Loss of volume of the affected lobe is uncommon during the acute pneumonic phase, but during resolution some collapse of the lobe is usual. Radiological opacities nearly always regress following the start of effective antibiotic therapy, but residual radiological change may persist for up to two or three months, although clearing is eventually complete in nearly all cases. Delayed resolution on the radiograph should always raise the possibility that the pneumonia may be the consequence of an underlying blockage of a bronchus, due to bronchial carcinoma, and is thus an indication for bronchoscopy. Pneumococcal pneumonia in patients with chronic bronchitis and emphysema may present as a bronchopneumonia. *Pleural effusion*, which is usually sterile with a predominance of polymorphs in the fluid, is an uncommon but well recognized late manifestation.

# Treatment

*Strep. pneumoniae* is nearly always sensitive to penicillin, and the usual regimen is to give one million units of benzylpenicillin twice daily intramuscularly for 48 hours, followed by 250 mg of phenoxymethyl-penicillin by mouth four times daily for a further seven to ten days. An alternative is ampicillin 250 mg four times daily for 10 days, which is as effective as penicillin. Central cyanosis, or an arterial $PO_2$ below 8.0 kPa (60 mmHg) is an indication for continuous oxygen therapy, most effectively given at a rate of 2 litres/minute by nasal prongs, which will be worn by the patient, and so raise the arterial $PO_2$ to normal levels, whereas most oxygen masks are discarded from time to time. Pleuritic pain should be relieved by 10–15 mg of morphine given intramuscularly six-hourly, for the first 24–48 hours, before the antibiotic treatment controls this symptom. This narcotic should only be withheld if the pneumonia is associated with carbon dioxide retention, and this will usually mean that the patient is a pre-existing sufferer from chronic bronchitis and emphysema. In the rare desperately ill patient, higher doses of antibiotics may be required, and if the aetiology is not clear and staphylococcal pneumonia is a possibility, it is reasonable to combine ampicillin 500 mg six-hourly by mouth with benzylpenicillin 10 megaunits daily intravenously and flucloxacillin 1 g six-hourly by mouth, thereby covering the possibilities that the patient is suffering from a pneumonia due to *Staph. pyogenes*, *Strep. pneumoniae*, or infection with both *Strep. pneumoniae* and *Haemophilus influenzae*.

If the patient is shocked, high doses of parenteral steroids may be used, although there is still controversy as to their value, for evidence from controlled trials is not available in these desperately ill patients. *Strep. pneumoniae* which are relatively resistant to penicillin have now been reported from Papua New Guinea, Canada, Britain and the United States. *Strep. pneumoniae* resistant to sulphonamides, tetracycline, erythromycin, lincomycin and chloramphenicol have also been described. *Strep. pneumoniae* resistant to penicillin in addition to these other antibiotics have been isolated in South Africa. These variant organisms have to date been very rare, but clearly the possibility of failure to respond to penicillin remains, so that full antibiotic sensitivity of the organisms should be determined if there is no response to treatment with penicillin or ampicillin within 48 hours.

# Staphylococcal pneumonia

## Epidemiology

Staphylococcal pneumonia is a major cause of death during an influenza epidemic, being a secondary invader in lungs which are already the seat of infection with influenza virus, this sequence being particularly common in patients with pre-existing chronic bronchitis and emphysema. Staphylococcal pneumonia is also a major cause of bacterial pneumonia in infancy. Recurrent staphylococcal infections are very frequent in the lungs of patients with cystic fibrosis (see Chapter 12). Staphylococcal pneumonia is also often encountered in debilitated hospital patients, often postoperatively following the use of wide spectrum antibiotics to which the invading staphylococcus is resistant.

## Pathology

Fulminating staphylococcal pneumonia causes haemorrhagic pulmonary oedema, but in less severe infections the pneumonia starts as consolidation in lobules and surrounding airways, with a marked tendency to *multiple abscess formation*, and subsequent development of thin-walled air spaces, *pneumatoceles* which can expand enormously, particularly in children. Pleural effusion is often a common complication, and this is often purulent, again particularly in children.

## Clinical features

A rapid onset with fever, central cyanosis and rapid grunting respiration are characteristic in infancy. This pattern is often also followed in the rare cases which occur in previously healthy adults, but they usually also complain of pleuritic chest pain. Hospital-acquired infections are often postoperative or in patients receiving steroids or antibiotics, fever, cough, purulent sputum with haemoptysis all being possible presenting features. The physical signs include those of consolidation, or merely coarse crepitations, or a pleural effusion may be the presenting feature. Staphylococcal pneumonia complicating chronic bronchitis and emphysema during an influenzal epidemic can cause a patient to be desperately ill, with severe central cyanosis; bronchial breathing is then rarely present, but shock with tachycardia, hypotension and cold extremities may be the presenting picture. Pneumatoceles can cause the mediastinum to shift away from the side of the lesion, and breath sounds are diminished over a pneumatocele, but there is a resonant percussion note, serving to distinguish this clinically from a pleural effusion.

## Radiology

The disease is usually bilateral in adults, with areas of consolidation often proceeding to multiple fluid-containing cavities, but in the adult these rarely form pneumatoceles as they resolve, although this is characteristic of staphylococcal pneumonia in children. Pleural effusion or empyema is common in staphylococcal pneumonia. Pneumonia occurring as part of a staphylococcal septicaemia, which has resulted from a primary staphylococcal infection elsewhere in the body, presents as multiple nodular opacities which may erode into air spaces, so causing cavities. In infancy, overt consolidation often precedes development of the thin-walled pneumatoceles, and these may occupy the whole of one side of the chest, and may simulate a tension pneumothorax. The production of pneumatoceles in an infant is almost pathognomonic of staphylococcal pneumonia, but pleural effusion is also a very common complication in children, and this may result from a staphylococcal empyema following the rupture of a staphylococcal cavity into the pleural space.

## Diagnosis

The radiographic features described above are very suggestive of staphylococcal pneumonia, but the diagnosis is confirmed by isolating a pure culture of staphylococci from the sputum. However, demonstration of multiple clumps of Gram-positive cocci in a Gram stain of the sputum should lead to specific treatment being started. Blood culture is often positive in severely affected patients, or where an empyema complicates a primary non-thoracic origin of the staphylococcal infection.

## Treatment

It is wise to assume that any staphylococcal infection is resistant to penicillin, and thus therapy should start with flucloxacillin (500 mg four times daily by mouth) combined with benzylpenicillin in a dose of at least 2 megaunits by intramuscular injection 12-hourly. The antibiotic sensitivity of the specific staphylococcus cannot be known for 24–48 hours when the results of cultures become available, and at that time the treatment may be adjusted depending on such sensitivities. In the patient with chronic bronchitis and emphysema, an infection with *Haemophilus influenzae* is also possible, and thus ampicillin (500 mg six-hourly by mouth) should be added to the initial treatment, as the third drug in addition to the flucloxacillin and benzylpenicillin. Chemotherapy is continued for at least 10 days. Arterial blood gas analysis should preferably precede the prescription of oxygen therapy, or of analgesics to relieve any pleuritic pain, for carbon dioxide retention may complicate staphylococcal pneumonia particularly in the patient with pre-existing chronic bronchitis and emphysema. Hypoxaemia combined with carbon dioxide retention (Type II respiratory failure, see Chapter 11) requires controlled oxygen therapy, and of course in such patients opiates should be avoided. However, staphylococcal pneumonia in such a patient with pre-existing chronic bronchitis and emphysema may be such a devastating illness that life-threatening respiratory acidosis persists despite controlled oxygen therapy, so that mechanical ventilation may be necessary (see Chapter 11).

# Klebsiella pneumonia

This serious Gram-negative bacillary pneumonia occurs most often in men who are over 60 years of age, and is particularly common in alcoholics. The mortality can be over 40%. Multiple lobar involvement, often including the upper lobes with diffuse exudates expanding the lobes, so that the fissures bulge outwards, often progresses to cavity formation.

*Clinically* the onset is often abrupt, with pleuritic pain, fever and severe breathlessness, with greenish blood-streaked sputum. The patient is often shocked at the time of presentation. Signs of consolidation may be present on examination of the chest, but there is rarely a very pronounced peripheral blood leucocytosis, and a low or normal white count is a bad prognostic sign, as polymorphonuclear leucocytes are essential to clearing of this pulmonary infection. The sputum smear often shown numerous Gram-negative bacilli and treatment must then start at once. Klebsiellae vary in their antibiotic sensitivity and this must be determined in each patient, but clearly therapy cannot await the result of sensitivity tests. In Britain, where chloramphenicol is rarely used for treating other conditions, experience suggests that chloramphenicol (2 g daily), combined with streptomycin (1–2 g intramuscularly daily), is often effective. This can then be followed by ampicillin or tetracycline, if the klebsiellae are found to be sensitive to these organisms. In North America a combination of gentamicin (1.5 mg/kg intravenously or intramuscularly eight-hourly), ampicillin (2 g intravenously four-hourly), or cephalosporin (1–2 g intravenously every four to six hours) is favoured. Such a regimen requires measurement of serum levels of gentamicin which should not be above 2 mg/litre in the trough, nor higher than 14 mg/litre at peak. Many of these severely ill patients have renal failure complicating the pneumonia, emphasizing the need for careful monitoring of gentamicin serum levels. Oxygen may be required in high concentrations to restore a normal arterial $PO_2$, and this can be safely given if, as is usual, the arterial $PCO_2$ is low. For the same reasons narcotic analgesics can be used to control pain without fear of inducing Type II respiratory failure with carbon dioxide retention. The shocked patient presents a serious problem, and if the low cardiac output of shock is combined with arterial hypoxaemia, it is obvious that tissue oxygenation will be very poor. High concentrations of oxygen ensure that the arterial $PO_2$ is maintained over 10–12 kPa, and possibly blood transfusion if the haemoglobin is below 12 g/dl, to ensure that the blood oxygen-carrying capacity is as high as possible, intravenous fluids controlled by monitoring the central venous pressure, and high doses of dexamethasone or hydrocortisone may all be needed. Nonetheless the prognosis is poor, and severe *Klebsiella* pneumonia is a recognized cause of the adult respiratory distress syndrome (see Chapter 11).

# Other bacterial lobar pneumonias

Tuberculosis is always a possible cause of apparent lobar pneumonia, tuberculous lobar pneumonia usually being of gradual onset, and the only certain way of excluding tuberculosis is by examination of sputum for acid fast bacilli in all cases of pneumonia.

*Streptococcus pyogenes* usually causes bronchopneumonia, but can closely mimic staphylococcal pneumonia, and may be a complication of measles.

Pneumonia due to *Pseudomonas aeruginosa* (a Gram-negative bacillus which can grow in some 'antiseptic' solutions, and is a common skin commensal) presents with a radiological pattern like staphylococcal pneumonia, often being a hospital-acquired infection in patients receiving multiple antibiotic and steroid therapy, or during mechanical ventilation through a tracheostomy tube where the organism may be acquired from contaminated humidifiers. Patients with impaired polymorphonuclear leucocyte responses are particularly at risk. The onset of *Pseudomonas* pneumonia may be abrupt with fever, restlessness, haemoptysis with green sputum, and often a relative bradycardia. Combination chemotherapy with gentamicin (1.5 mg/kg intramuscularly eight-hourly) and intravenous carbenicillin (5 g four-hourly) is indicated for patients with obvious systemic infection. Again, as with *Klebsiella* pneumonia treated with gentamicin, dosage should be monitored by serum levels. Tobramycin in a dose of 3 mg/kg/day intramuscularly eight-hourly appears to be more effective than gentamicin against many stains of *Pseudomonas*. As with gentamicin, 8th nerve toxicity is recognized, and the dose should be modified in patients with impaired renal function. Even if this is normal, a maximal dose of 5 mg/kg/day should not be exceeded. Serum concentrations of tobramycin over 12 mg/litre should be avoided and powerful diuretics should not be given at the same time.

The mere finding of *Pseudomonas* in sputum or tracheal swabs, without evidence of systemic infection, suggests that it is merely acting as a commensal in these sites, and thus specific antibiotic therapy may not be indicated.

# Bronchopneumonia

In patients with an acute infective exacerbation of pre-existing chronic bronchitis and emphysema, infection with *Streptococcus pneumoniae* and *Haemophilus influenzae* is very common, the infection spreading from the bronchi to the terminal air spaces, usually producing bilateral patchy opacities which are often more prominent at the bases. This pattern is termed bronchopneumonia. The patient may complain of increasing breathlessness, with cough and purulent sputum and physical examination shows the hyperinflated chest characteristic of chronic bronchitis and emphysema, bilateral rhonchi, and occasionally basal coarse crepitations. Bronchial breathing is rare. Central cyanosis is usually prominent when the patient is breathing air, and there may be signs of carbon dioxide retention, as in the distended forearm veins, a flapping tremor of the outstretched hands and tachycardia. Arterial blood gas analysis confirms the presence of Type II respiratory failure, hypoxaemia being combined with carbon dioxide retention and respiratory acidosis, which is usually of the acute-on-chronic type (see Chapters 3 and 11). Ampicillin (500 mg four times daily by mouth) for ten days nearly always controls pneumococcal and *H. influenzae* infection, but in an influenza epidemic (due to influenza virus) where the patient is desperately ill, it is also wise to assume that he may have a staphylococcal pneumonia, and so add penicillin and flucloxacillin as described above, at least until bacterial cultures of the sputum are available. Controlled oxygen therapy (see Chapter 11) may be required, along with bronchodilators and diuretics.

# Mycoplasma pneumonia

The commonest non-bacterial cause for pneumonia is an infection with *Mycoplasma pneumoniae*, a small organism which lacks a rigid cell wall, and is about 150 μm in diameter, similar to that of a medium sized virus. *Mycoplasma* multiply on the surface of cells in the respiratory tract, inhibiting mucociliary clearance, and eventually killing the epithelial cells locally. The organism resists phagocytosis by polymorphonuclear leucocytes. It is not firmly adsorbed to the polymorph surface, except in the presence of antibody, when phagocytosis and killing occur.

The disease tends to have a peak incidence in the community every few years, particularly in young adults, but major epidemics similar to influenza A virus are very uncommon.

## Clinical features and investigations

Fever is usually low-grade, and can last for two or three weeks, with a non-productive cough which is usually associated with headache, malaise, muscular aches, but with few direct respiratory symptoms apart from occasional retrosternal chest pain. Pleuritic pain is uncommon. Examination of the chest rarely reveals abnormal physical signs, apart from crepitations, but on occasion the disease may clinically mimic lobar pneumonia.

The white cell count is usually normal; the ESR is high, and specific Ig antibodies are prominent. These act as cold agglutinins, and may rarely lead to a haemolytic anaemia. A four-fold rise in specific antibody titre over a ten-day period is usually regarded as diagnostic of mycoplasma infection, being more specific than the mere demonstration of cold agglutinins. Culture of *Mycoplasma pneumoniae* takes two to 12 weeks and is so of little use in clinical practice.

## Radiology

A fine reticular pattern, which can be unilateral or bilateral, and which may later progress to patchy consolidation taking up to six weeks to clear, usually distinguishes *Mycoplasma pneumonia* from bacterial pneumonia. Lower lobe involvement is more common, and hilar gland involvement is usually confined to children. Pleural effusion is rare.

## Treatment

Tetracycline (500 mg six-hourly by mouth) or erythromycin (250 mg six-hourly by mouth) are the drugs of choice. *Mycoplasma* does not respond to the penicillins.

# Legionnaire's disease

## Epidemiology

In the autumn of 1976 4500 American ex-servicemen attended their annual convention in Philadelphia, many of them staying in the Belview Stratford Hotel. There were some 200 cases of serious respiratory disease, with 29 deaths. Brilliant scientific detective work at the Centre for Disease Control in Atlanta led to the isolation of a previously unknown organism (*Legionella pneumophila*), subsequently proved to be the cause of pneumonia even in 1947, and now thought to account for up to 10% of all cases of otherwise undiagnosed pneumonia. Similar epidemics amongst previously fit subjects have occurred from 1965, including an outbreak in tourists visiting Spain in 1973 and 1980. Sporadic outbreaks have also occurred in previously healthy travellers, and this can lead to sporadic community-acquired infection, as in Nottingham, England, where 1.5% of the population had serological evidence of previous *Legionella* infection. Hospital-associated infection can occur in immune compromised patients. Person-to-person spread does not seem to occur, but the organism is widespread in soil and contaminates water cooling systems and may lurk in shower fittings.

## Pathology

Acute pneumonia is associated with multiple lobar consolidation, which can progress to organizing pneumonia, with intense inflammation being followed by fibrosis. Abscess formation has been observed. The organism is only detectable by complicated stains, including silver preparations, and is very difficult to culture. The clinical diagnosis is confirmed by serology.

## Clinical features

After an incubation period of two to ten days, the patient develops malaise, muscle pains and fever with cough, but little sputum production although haemoptysis is recognized. Nausea, vomiting or diarrhoea is present in at least 50% of acute cases. Breathlessness progresses, rigors and confusion sometimes leading to a well recognized encephalopathic picture.

Consolidation may be unilateral and lobar in distribution at first, but often progresses to show multilobular radiographic opacities, despite therapy with penicillin. Pleural effusion is sometimes associated. Laboratory clues to the diagnosis include hyponatraemia, a modest elevation of liver enzymes, moderate polymorph leucocytosis, and in some cases microscopic haematuria. Disseminated intravascular coagulation has been recorded. Culture of sputum yields no conventional organisms.

The diagnosis can thus be suspected in a patient who has a prodromal 'viral illness'; dry cough *or* confusion *or* diarrhoea; lymphopenia without neutropenia; or hyponatraemia. Diagnostic confirmation depends upon an indirect fluorescent antibody test.

## Treatment

Erythromycin is the drug of choice, given as 500 mg either intravenously or orally six-hourly. The organism is also sensitive to rifampicin and in some cases tetracycline. Relapse has been described after two weeks of erythromycin, and it is probable that therapy should continue for at least one month. Over half of the survivors from the 1976 epidemic still had impaired respiratory function over two years later.

# Virus pneumonia

Pneumonia is recognized as either a primary event or a complication of the following virus infection:

1. *Adenoviruses*, particularly common in military recruits.

2. *Respiratory syncitial virus (RSV)* with bronchiolitis within the first six months of life and pneumonia in later infancy.

3. *Coxsackie and echoviruses*, sometimes associated with pleurodynia.

4. *Varicella*, where pnemonia is commoner in adults affected with chickenpox, and particularly in pregnancy when older children have chickenpox.

5. *Infectious mononucleosis*, when it is sometimes associated with pleural effusion.

The clinical features of these viral pneumonias are very similar to those of *Mycoplasma* pneumonia as described above. The diagnosis is usually made retrospectively by a four-fold rise in specific antibody titres in the serum, but rapid verification of the diagnosis can sometimes be obtained by expert examination of nasal washings by appropriate virological techniques. No specific therapy is available for virus pneumonia.

# Chlamydial pneumonia

Ornithosis (psittacosis) is an acute illness due to infection by *Chlamydia psittaci*, an intracellular parasite with a bacteria-like cell wall, which cannot grow outside an animal cell. After an incubation period of 7–14 days there is either an acute or slow onset of fever, malaise, myalgia, cough and sometimes blood-tinged sputum. Confusion and delirium may occur, and cyanosis is common. As with *Mycoplasm* pneumonia bilateral crepitations may be present, but consolidation is uncommon, and the radiograph shows an interstitial pneumonia which may be apparently widespread. Hepatosplenomegaly, pericarditis and myocarditis are all recognized complications. The diagnosis is confirmed either by a rise in antibody response or by isolation of *C. psittaci* from blood or sputum, in cell culture techniques. Tetracycline (500 mg four times a day for adults) for 10 days is the treatment of choice.

# Pneumonia from uncommon infective agents

*Anthrax* can be contracted from unfinished wool, furs and hides which are contaminated with spores. Inhalation usually produces a fatal pneumonia, with high fever and shock, although this Gram-positive bacillus is very sensitive to penicillin. Pneumonic consolidation and a pleural effusion (which may be blood-stained) can be seen on the radiograph, often with hilar adenopathy.

*Brucellosis* is a rare cause of bronchopneumonia, lung abscess, empyema and hilar adenopathy.

*Listeriosis* can be acquired from animals, birds, milk and meat or from asymptomatic human carriers. Meningitis, septicaemia and endocarditis all occur, but pneumonia is a rare complication.

*Tularaemia*, from a Gram-negative organism, arises from contact with infected animals or their pelts. The pneumonia can be lobar or patchy infiltrates leading eventually to fibrosis. Hilar adenopathy, pleural effusions and empyema can result.

*Melioidosis* arises from contaminated dust or soil, and is endemic in south-east Asia. Radiologically the appearances are similar to tuberculosis, with cavities in the upper lobes, but an acute febrile pneumonia is also seen.

*Pneumonic plague* arises in endemic areas of Asia, Africa and South America. Haemoptysis and high fever of abrupt onset may be associated with widespread purpura — the Black Death of the Middle Ages. The chest radiograph shows rapid progression of the initial consolidation.

*Measles and whooping cough* can both cause pneumonia, which both clinically and radiologically can be very difficult to distinguish from a secondary bacterial pneumonia. Pathologically measles causes a giant cell pneumonia, which may give a diffuse reticular pattern on the chest radiograph.

# Pneumonia in the immune-compromised host

Therapeutic suppression of the immune system with steroids and/or cytotoxic agents is widely used today in the treatment of neoplastic disease (leukaemia, lymphomas and solid tumours) and also to prevent the rejection of transplanted organs. Hospital-acquired pneumonia is relatively common in such patients and may well be lethal unless specific therapy is rapidly instituted. Symptoms can include cough, breathlessness and fever, but the diagnosis is usually suspected when the chest radiograph shows an infiltrate which may be either a diffuse bilateral reticulonodular pattern or a localized lesion of lobar distribution. Such radiographic appearances in an immune-compromised patient can result from:

1. *Opportunistic infection*, which may be due to *Pneumocystis carinii* (see below), particularly in patients with leukaemia; *Aspergillus fumigatus*, invasive aspergillosis often presenting as a haemorrhagic pulmonary infarction, but with no diagnostic pattern on the chest radiograph; *Cryptococcus neoformans*, with pulmonary involvement as part of a disseminated infection; or *Candida albicans*, where again the lungs are often involved in a disseminated infection. Common *bacterial pathogens* in the immune-compromised host include pseudomonas, Klebsiellae, *E. coli*, and of course *Mycobacterium tuberculosis*. *Viral agents*, either alone or often in combination with *Pneumocystis* infection, include herpes simplex, cytomegalovirus, and the varicella–zoster virus. *Legionella pneumophila* can also cause pneumonia in the immune-compromised host.

2. *Pulmonary toxicity* from the cytotoxic drugs themselves (e.g. busulphan, bleomycin) or from radiotherapy involving the lung fields.

3. Extension (leukaemic infiltration, metastases from solid tumours) or a complication (e.g. bleeding from thrombocytopenia) of the *primary disease process*.

Opportunistic infection is a condition most likely to yield to successful treatment in these desperately ill patients, but isolation of the specific pathogen is often difficult. These patients rarely produce sputum, but invasive techniques such as transtracheal aspiration, transthoracic needle aspiration, and transbronchial biopsy with the fibreoptic bronchoscope, all carry a definite risk of serious bleeding as these patients are often thrombocytopenic. Open lung biopsy, which may well yield the definitive diagnosis by proving that lung tissue is invaded by one of these pathogens, will often be excluded by the severity of the respiratory failure complicating the pneumonia. Fibreoptic bronchoscopy, *without* transbronchial lung biopsy, but relying on bronchial brushings and washings, has been claimed to yield diagnostic material in up to 70% of such cases.

*Tuberculosis* is always a potential (and curable) cause of infection in the immune-compromised patient, in whom the disease may be rapidly progressive. All such patients should thus have a tuberculin skin test, chest radiograph and examination of the sputum for *Myco. tuberculosis* before starting their immunosuppressive regimen. If the tuberculin test is positive, or the radiograph shows 'old' calcified tuberculous lesions, including glands, chemoprophylaxis with isoniazid 300 mg/day should be given during immunosuppression.

*Pneumocystis carinii* is a protozoal parasite, existing as a cyst of 5–12 $\mu$m in diameter, containing four to eight trophozoites which are released as the mature cyst ruptures. Pneumonic infection presents with a non-productive cough and breathlessness, but only some half of these patients will have fever. Central cyanosis is usual and arterial hypoxaemia combined with a low $P\text{CO}_2$ is characteristic. The chest radiograph usually shows bilaterally symmetrical alveolar exudates, which appear to spread from the hilum and may eventually show an air bronchogram. A normal chest radiograph does not exclude the disease. The diagnosis depends upon demonstration of the characteristic cysts in tissue as obtained at fibreoptic bronchoscopy. Histological specimens may also show alveoli to be filled with a foamy eosinophilic exudate of trophozoites or cysts in the alveolar space.

Platelet transfusions can correct thrombocytopenia for a long enough period to allow the diagnostic transbronchial biopsy to be made. However, the diagnosis is often only considered after such an immune-compromised patient has failed to respond to 48–72 hours of antibacterial chemotherapy for an apparent pneumonic infection. *Pneumocystis* pneumonia responds to high doses of co-trimoxazole 14–18 tablets/day in the adult (20 mg trimethoprim and 100 mg sulphamethoxazole/kg/day) or parenterally, in the seriously ill patient, with modification of the dose in renal failure. Pentamidine isethionate, which was previously used for this infection, was effective but highly toxic.

Mycotic or opportunistic infections (*invasive aspergillosis* or *cryptococcosis*) require treatment with *amphotericin B*. This is given daily by intravenous infusion in dextrose, over six hours, in an initial dose of 0.25 mg/kg/day after a test dose of 1 mg intravenously. The dose is slowly increased to 1.0 mg/kg/day, to a maximum dosage of 1.5 mg/kg/day in a patient whose life is threatened by the mycotic infection. The total dose should normally be 2–4 g, rarely 5 g, and achieved over one to two months. Side effects are usually encountered with amphotericin B. Fever, chills, nausea, vomiting and abdominal pain can be prevented by analgesics. Most patients on higher doses develop reversible renal failure so that the daily dose must be halved if the serum creatinine level rises over 2 mg/dl. Potassium and magnesium can be lost from the body. A normochromic anaemia results from reversible bone marrow depression during treatment.

*Flucytosine* is added to amphotericin B in treating life-threatening cryptococcal infections, the dose of flucytosine again depending upon renal function.

# Aspiration pneumonia

Some oronasal secretions are inhaled in health, but patients are most at risk of developing pneumonia from aspiration when the cough mechanism is either impaired or overwhelmed. This can occur in the unconscious patient, in those with lower cranial nerve palsies, with dysphagia, protracted vomiting, or following use of a nasogastric tube, or an endotracheal tube.

In *chemical pneumonitis*, the lung inflammation is not initiated by infection, but results from aspiration of gastric acid (Mendelson's syndrome), or mineral oils such as petrol. Gastric acid inhalation (first described in women in labour) destroys the bronchial epithelium with resultant pulmonary oedema, atelectasis and haemorrhage, if the pH of the aspirate is below 3.0. As in other conditions causing the adult respiratory distress syndrome (see Chapter 11), this is associated with hypoxaemia, stiff lungs and widespread alveolar opacities on the radiograph and can sometimes lead eventually to pulmonary fibrosis. A sudden onset of wheeze and cyanosis in labour is characteristic. Treatment requires high concentrations of oxygen, with mechanical ventilation using positive end expiratory pressure (PEEP), if simpler measures do not relieve the hypoxaemia. Massive parenteral doses of steroids may be helpful if given early, within the first 12 hours, but antibiotics are probably of little value.

*Aspiration of inert liquids* (water, saline, blood and gastric contents with pH over 3.0) causes closure of small airways with resultant hypoxaemia, the closure being mediated by a vagal reflex. The inhalation of massive volumes of such fluids floods the alveoli (as in drowning), when tracheal suction is urgently required to save life.

*Inhalation of a foreign body* (see Fig. 40), a hazard particularly in young children, can cause few symptoms at the time, apart from cough, but later produces collapse behind the block if a segmental bronchus is obstructed, as then collateral ventilation cannot prevent the collapse. A bacterial pneumonia follows in a few weeks. Rarely a check valve mechanism causes local obstructive emphysema. Removal of the foreign body is an indication for a rigid bronchoscopy. The 'café coronary', when sudden dyspnoea, aphonia, and cyanosis leads rapidly to death at the dining table, usually arises from a chunk of ill-chewed steak obstructing the larynx.

A *bacterial aspiration pneumonia* should always be considered when a patient who is at risk (see above) develops a fever or leucocytosis. Clearly the unconscious patient will not complain of breathlessness and cough, nor will he raise purulent sputum. The chest radiograph shows patchy bronchopneumonic infiltration in those lobes that are lowest in that patient's position, e.g. posterior segments of the upper lobe and apical segments of the lower lobes when the patient is supine, but lower lobes in the upright patient. Often pathogens are obtained only by transtracheal aspiration or fibreoptic bronchoscopy, preferably using a sheathed sampling catheter, or from a pleural effusion. *Anaerobic organisms* are common but will be missed unless special culture methods are used. The infection is commonly mixed *Strep. pneumoniae* and *Staph. aureus* being the common aerobic organisms; the additional anaerobic organisms are similar to the usual mouth commensals. If untreated, an aspiration pneumonia can lead to a lung abscess, empyema or necrotising pneumonia. Treatment by intramuscular benzylpenicillin (4 megaunits daily for uncomplicated cases, rising to 10 megaunits daily for lung abscess) is often effective, as the antibacterial spectrum of penicillin includes the common anaerobic organisms. However, metronidazole 400 mg orally three times daily, is often added, as it is specifically active against *Bacillus fragilis*, which is resistant to penicillin. Empyema may require rib resection to provide adequate drainage, in addition to the antibacterial chemotherapy.

*Chronic destructive pneumonia*, often in one upper lobe, has recently been described in African men who present with chest pain, haemoptysis and foul-smelling sputum. Consolidation, lung fibrosis and bronchiectasis are often found with pus-filled cavities containing both aerobic and anaerobic bacteria. Again the anaerobic bacteria are those species commonly found as mouth commensals, indicating that the condition results from chronic aspiration. Metronidazole in combination with cephalosporins and benzylpenicillin has been shown to be the best treatment for this potentially lethal condition.

# The diagnostic approach to pneumonia

Pneumonia may be confused with other conditions presenting with similar clinical features. These include:

1. *Chest pain of sudden onset* is typical of myocardial infarction, where the pain is central, is very rarely related to breathing, and usually radiates to the arms and/or throat; or of a dissecting aneurysm

of the aorta, and rarely pericarditis or mediastinitis, where again the pain is not pleuritic in nature.

2. *Other causes of sudden pleuritic pain* include pulmonary infarction, often associated with breathlessness, sometimes with haemoptysis, but the initial sputum is rarely purulent and fever is not prominent. Secondary infection of an infarct may make recognition of the primary event very difficult, but a clue may be given by finding a source for a pulmonary embolus, ECG changes of right heart strain, and possibly an elevated jugular venous pressure. Arterial hypoxaemia with a low $P_{CO_2}$ is characteristic of both conditions, and a lung scan in pneumonia is probably very similar to that in pulmonary infarction, but a reduced local perfusion in a region of the lung, yet with preservation of normal ventilation without an obvious radiological opacity in that region, strongly favours embolism. However, rapidly reversible perfusion defects are also seen in bronchial asthma, but this of course can be excluded by finding a normal $FEV_1$ before the scan is carried out.

3. *Spontaneous pneumothorax*, with chest pain of pleuritic nature, is usually readily distinguished by physical signs, with absent breath sounds and diminished movement on the affected side. The chest radiograph is usually diagnostic. A *fractured rib* as a cause of pleuritic pain is unlikely to be associated with fever, unless of course the diminished movement on the affected side resulting from the pain causes local atelectasis, possibly with a superadded infection.

4. *Other causes of sudden breathlessness* include bronchial asthma, pulmonary oedema (possibly complicating myocardial infarction), sudden occlusion of an airway by a foreign body, allergic alveolitis or, of course, spontaneous pneumothorax or pulmonary embolism.

5. *Other causes of fever of sudden onset* possibly with rigors include septicaemia, and particularly urinary tract infections. Fever of slower onset, as occurring in pneumonia in the postoperative patient or immune-compromised host, clearly has many other causes, including tuberculosis, disseminated carcinoma (particularly hypernephroma), leukaemia or reticuloses and in the postoperative patient localized collections of pus as in a subphrenic abscess.

6. *Bronchial carcinoma* is an important cause of secondary pneumonia, with 'infection behind the block'. Delayed resolution of an apparently simple bacterial pneumonia in a smoker should always lead to consideration of this possibility. If clubbing of the fingers is present, or if a pneumonia resolves slowly, or if the radiograph shows partial or complete lobar or segmental collapse, bronchoscopy should not be delayed.

7. *Bronchiectasis* may well lead to recurrent episodes of pneumonia with pleuritic pain, but the long history of persistent purulent sputum or haemoptysis, with clubbing of the fingers and persistent crepitations, may give evidence of the true diagnosis, which can be

confirmed by bronchography. An inhaled foreign body can cause recurrent episodes of pneumonia, again with 'infection behind the block'.

8. *Allergic alveolitis*, following acute exposure to heavy doses of an appropriate antigen, can mimic a viral pneumonia with breathlessness associated with myalgia and fever. However, a history of antigen exposure usually provides the clue, although radiographic opacities mimicking pneumonia may occur. Allergic bronchopulmonary aspergillosis causing mucus impaction, with radiographic opacities, and breathlessness, may also rarely mimic pneumonia.

A clinical diagnosis of pneumonia is of course incomplete without an attempt to *identify the causal agent*. This is often obtained from examining the Gram stain of sputum, but culture may be necessary, and no organism may be found if antimicrobial agents have already been used. Purulent sputum without organisms may be due to sputum eosinophilia, as in bronchopulmonary aspergillosis. Viral pneumonia, or pneumonia due to *Mycoplasma* or *Chlamydia* may depend upon a rise in antibody titres in serum for diagnosis. Sputum may not be produced in the unconscious or in the immune-compromised and bronchoscopic techniques may be necessary to obtain the causal organism. In the ill patient without evidence of a causal organism from the sputum examination, therapy is often empirical, based upon the diagnostic possibilities in that clinical circumstance. If the patient is desperately ill it is wise to consider the range of organisms which could have produced the clinical condition, and treat appropriately. Such therapy may include penicillin, flucloxacillin and ampicillin, covering together the possibility of *Strep. pneumoniae, H. influenzae, Staph. aureus*; chloramphenicol and streptomycin if *Klebsiella* is a possibility (or gentamicin plus a cephalosporin); streptomycin and isoniazid which would cover the possibility of tuberculous pneumonia; and erythromycin to deal with *Legionella pneumophila*, and possibly mycoplasmal infection. Such polypharmacy clearly carries much risk of drug interactions and side effects, but may at some times be justifiable for initial treatment in a desperately ill patient, in whom proof (or exclusion) of the nature of the microbiological agent causing the pneumonia will not be available for 24–48 hours. When this does become clear, obviously only the specific antibiotics should be continued.

Most patients with pneumonia in whom a microbiological diagnosis is not established will nonetheless respond to penicillin or ampicillin, but it must be emphasized that most cases of clinical pneumonia result from *Strep. pneumoniae* infection. Even though the organism cannot be observed in sputum, evidence of such infection may be confirmed later by a rise in pneumococcal antigen or antibodies in the sputum or serum. However in any case of pneumonia the diagnosis should be reviewed if there is no clinical response to therapy within 48 hours.

# Further reading

AUSTRIAN, R. (1977) Pneumococcal infection and pneumococcal vaccine. *New Engl. J. Med.*, **297**, 938–939.

BALOWS, A. and FRASER, D. W. (1979) International symposium on legionnaires' disease. *Ann. intern. Med.*, **90**, 489–703.

BARTLETT, J. G. (1979) Anaerobic bacterial pneumonitis. *Am. Rev. resp. Dis.*, **119**, 19–23

CAMERON, I. R. and PHILIPS, I. (1980) Pneumonia. In *Recent Advances in Respiratory Medicine II*, ed. D. C. Flenley. Edinburgh: Churchill Livingstone.

KIRKPATRICK, C. H. and RENOLDS, H. Y. Editors (1976) *Lung Biology in Health and Disease, 1. Immunologic and Infectious Reactions in the Lung.* New York and Basel: Marcel Dekker

LEVINE, D. P. and LERNER, A. M. (1978) The clinical spectrum of *Mycoplasma pneumoniae* infections. *Med. Clins N. Am.*, **62**(5), 961–978.

MIMS, C. A. (1977) *The Pathogenesis of Infectious Disease.* London: Academic Press.

PUTNAM, J. S. and TUAZON, C. (1980) Symposium on infectious lung diseases. *Med. Clins N. Am.*, **64**, no. 3.

SCHMID, R. E., ANHALT, J. P., WOLD, A. D. et al. (1979) Sputum counter-immunoelectrophoresis in the diagnosis of pneumococcal pneumonia. *Am. Rev. resp. Dis.*, **119**, 345–348.

SINGER, C., ARMSTRONG, D., ROSEN, P. P., WALZER, P. D. and YU, B. (1979) Diffuse pulmonary infiltrates in immunosuppressed patients. *Am. J. Med.*, **66**, 110–120.

WILLIAMS, D. M., KRICK, J. A. and REMINGTON, J. S. (1976) Pulmonary infection in the compromised host, Parts I and II. *Am. Rev. resp. Dis.*, **114**, 359–394, 593–627.

WYNNE, J. W. and MODELL, J. H. (1977) Respiratory aspiration of stomach contents. *Ann. intern. Med.*, **87**, 466–474.

YOSHIKAWA, T. T., CHOW, A. W. and GUZE, L. B. (1980) *Infectious Diseases: Diagnosis and Management.* Boston: Houghton Mifflin.

# 9

# Chronic Bronchitis and Emphysema

*Chronic bronchitis* is defined as an increase in mucus production by the lower respiratory tract, presenting clinically as persistent cough with sputum production for more than three months in each year over the previous three years. *Emphysema*, in contrast, is defined pathologically as a dilatation of the air spaces lying beyond the terminal bronchioles of the lungs, with destruction of their walls. The two conditions, chronic bronchitis and emphysema, are nearly always associated in any individual patient and it is now recognized that they cannot be clearly distinguished from each other in life. In this chapter therefore they will always be referred to as a single entity 'chronic bronchitis and emphysema'.

## Epidemiology

Chronic bronchitis and enphysema is the commonest cause of loss of work in Britain, accounting for the vast majority of the 30 million working days lost each year in Britain from chronic respiratory disease. It is far commoner in men and a survey amongst representative general practices throughout Britain in 1961 showed that 17% of all men and 8% of all women aged between 40 and 64 years had clinical symptoms of chronic bronchitis and emphysema. The incidence in England is probably highest in the world, Scotland probably being second, and in both countries the disease has its highest incidence in the major centres of industry, the Midlands, northern Britain and the midland valley of Scotland. It is rare in life-long non-smokers and shows a greater predominance in socio-economic classes 4 and 5 (manual and unskilled workers) than can be accounted for entirely on the basis of the difference in smoking habits between the socio-economic classes. The complicated disease, with chronic hypoxaemia and cor pulmonale (the 'blue and bloated' syndrome; see later), is probably commoner in Britain than in North America, but chronic bronchitis and emphysema occurs throughout the world, being particularly frequent in industrial populations, including those in Asia and China. An acute exacerbation of chronic bronchitis and emphysema is one of the commonest causes of acute medical admission to hospital during the British winter. The disease often shows an inexorable progression, with progressive breathlessness ultimately leading to early retirement, followed by increasing restriction of daily activities, and eventually death from cor pulmonale or respiratory failure some 10–20 years after the first symptoms.

*Known risk factors*, which indicate an increased incidence of the disease, thus include cigarette smoking, low socio-economic class, male sex, bronchial hyper-reactivity with or without atopy (see Chapter 10), repeated respiratory infections in infancy and childhood, and existence of another family member with the disease.

# Pathology

*Chronic bronchitis* is associated with hypertrophy of the mucous glands of the tracheobronchial tree, so that goblet cells (see Chapter 1) spread distally, being found in the terminal bronchioles where they are not present in health. The submucosal glands of the trachea and major bronchi are also greatly enlarged in both number and size of the cells, the resultant ratio of the thickness of this glandular layer to the thickness of the whole bronchial wall (the gland/wall or Reid ratio) being over 30–35%. The mucus produced not only is excessive in quantity, but also tends to be more viscid, from changes in the glycoprotein molecules. Small patchy areas of atelectasis and bronchiectasis are widespread in the lungs, particularly in patients who have died in an acute exacerbation of respiratory failure due to chronic bronchitis and emphysema. The sputum is usually infected in such patients, the commonest pathogens being *Haemophilus influenzae* and *Strep. pneumoniae*.

*Emphysema* may be centrilobular or panacinar (Fig. 42). The centrilobular form, where the centre of the affected lobule is destroyed, is most prominent in the upper zones of a vertical cut slice of the whole lung (Fig. 42). In panacinar emphysema most of the alveoli forming the normal lung acinus are destroyed, with only a few vascular strands crossing these spaces. Panacinar emphysema is usually predominantly in the lower lobes.

Right ventricular hypertrophy, an increase in the amount of smooth muscle in the walls of the pulmonary arterioles and doubling of the elastic lamina of these vessels are all characteristic pathological features of the pulmonary hypertension which is associated with cor pulmonale in this disease. Right ventricular hypertrophy is shown by an increase in the weight of the right ventricle, when dissected free from the left ventricle and septum, as shown by the ratio of these two weights (Fulton ratio) being less than 2.0.

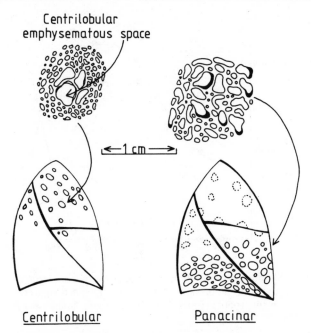

*Fig. 42.*   Pathological appearances within the acini of centrilobular emphysema (left-hand) and panacinar emphysema (right-hand). Centrilobular emphysema is usually mostly in the upper lobes and the apex of the lower lobes, whereas panacinar emphysema may be predominantly basal in the rare alpha-1-antitrypsin deficiency or can be widespread throughout the lung fields

## Pathogenesis

Cigarette smoke contains over 1200 distinct chemicals which include aldehydes, hydrogen cyanide, hydrogen sulphide, mercury and many complex organic molecules including benzpyrene, a potent carcinogen (Fig. 43). Carbon monoxide is also present, British cigarettes each yielding between 10 and 20 mg of carbon monoxide. Animal studies have shown that prolonged exposure to cigarette smoke can provoke hyperplasia of the mucous glands, and similar effects result from sulphur dioxide, which is a common atmospheric pollutant in smoky industrial cities. Sulphur dioxide and the particulates of cigarette smoke cause bronchoconstriction from stimulation of bronchial irritant receptors. This bronchoconstriction can be blocked by atropine, showing that it depends upon a vagal reflex. These bronchoconstrictor responses are all more marked in heavy cigarette smokers in whom airway muscle is hypertrophied. Thus, irritation of

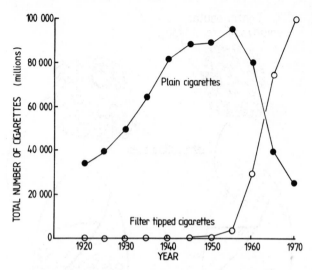

*Fig. 43.*    Annual consumption of cigarettes in the United Kingdom, showing the marked change to filter-tipped cigarettes occurring in the 1960s. (*From J. M. Wald (1976) Lancet, 1, 136*)

the bronchial tree by either cigarette smoke or chemical industrial pollutants increases mucus production, with hypertrophy of the mucous glands, and also leads to hypertrophy of the bronchial smooth muscle. Both contribute to the airways obstruction which characterizes chronic bronchitis.

The pathogenesis of panacinar and centrilobular emphysema has become much clearer in the last few years. In 1962 Swedish workers showed that a deficiency of a normal constituent of plasma proteins, *alpha-1-antitrypsin* was associated with bilateral basal panacinar emphysema, presenting in men under the age of 40 years. About the same time American workers showed that emphysema could be induced experimentally in animals by instillation of papain (a proteolytic enzyme from plants), into the trachea. These two observations have led to the *proteolytic theory* of the pathogenesis of emphysema (Fig. 44). Smoking causes the pulmonary alveolar macrophages, a major defence cell of the respiratory tract, to accumulate around the terminal bronchioles. In smokers these macrophages are abnormal, being pigmented, with blunting of their normal finely ruffled cell membrane, and they more readily release their endogenous proteolytic enzymes than do pulmonary alveolar macrophages from non-smokers. It is thus proposed that smoking damages macrophages so that they do indeed release these enzymes, thus digesting lung tissue locally. In

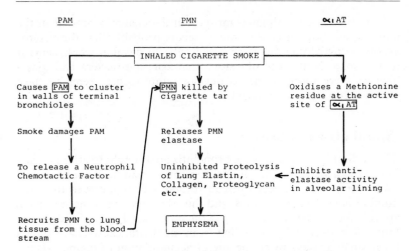

*Fig. 44.*    The proteolytic theory of the pathogenesis of emphysema. The three principal factors concerned are: PAM, pulmonary alveolar macrophages; PMN, polymorphonuclear leucocytes; AT, alpha$_1$ antitrypsin. (*After Crystal 1981*)

addition a powerful proteolytic enzyme is released from dying polymorphonuclear leucocytes (PMN), which are of course attracted to the lungs from the blood stream to die in their phagocytic battle in episodes of bacterial pulmonary infection, as evidenced by purulence of the sputum.

The defence against this ever-present threat of endogenous digestion by these enzymes lies in the serum alpha-1-antitrypsin, also a normal constituent of airway lining fluids. However, cigarette smoke has a powerful oxidant action, so tending to inactivate the antiproteolytic action of the alpha-1-antitrypsin. Similar oxidants are released by the dying PMN. There is thus a dynamic equilibrium between the burden of proteolytic enzyme release from pulmonary alveolar macrophages and polymorphonuclear leucocytes in smokers, which is normally opposed by the alpha-1-antitrypsin. In established cigarette smokers this balance is swung towards an increase in proteolytic activity, with the resultant digestion of the lung acini resulting in centrilobular emphysema. In contrast, the panacinar emphysema of the *rare alpha-1-antitrypsin-deficient patient* seems to arise from the unopposed action of elastase secreted from polymorphonuclear leucocytes, which are sequestered from the blood stream and not from the airway, so accounting for the difference in anatomical pattern of panacinar emphysema as opposed to centrilobular emphysema.

Clinically evident alpha-1-antitrypsin deficiency is present in the homozygous patient (PiZZ) but it seems probable that the hetero-zygotes (PiMZ) may be more susceptible to develop emphysema if they smoke. Sadly, the old story that bagpipe players and glass-blowers were more prone to develop emphysema seems to have returned to Celtic mythology!

### 'Small airways disease'

The earliest lesions of chronic bronchitis are thought to arise patchily in the small airways of the lungs, less than 2 mm in diameter, where such lesions may be very difficult to detect in life, due to the large number of such small airways, and thus the very large cross-sectional area of all the small airways within the lungs (see Fig. 3). Study of the lungs of smokers who have died from incidental causes have shown these small airways to be the site of accumulation of pigment-laden pulmonary alveolar macrophages, goblet cell metaplasia, and squa-mous cell metaplasia of the normal columnar ciliated epithelium (see Chapter 1) with patchy ulceration and inflammatory cell infiltrates. These changes are thought to interfere with the production of surfactant in small airways so that they become mechanically unstable, and so close readily. Sophisticated tests of lung function — comparison of the flow–volume curves (see Fig. 5) breathing air with those breathing 80% helium (lower density); an increase in the closing volume (see Fig. 11); and development of frequency dependence of compliance (whereby the lungs appear to become stiffer as the breathing rate increases) — may all be physiological indications of abnormalities in these small airways in life (see Chapter 1). Abnormality in these sophisticated functional tests may be present before the patient has a reduction in $FEV_1$, as this latter probably reflects changes in the larger airways. However, it must be stressed that the hypothesis that future disabling chronic bronchitis and emphysema starts in the small airways, where it can be detected by these tests in life, yet remains to be proved.

# Clinical features

*Cough* occurs at first only in the morning, many smokers being surprised to learn that their 'smoker's cough' is abnormal. Cough is usually productive of at first a mucoid sputum, which becomes purulent in an exacerbation, when *H. influenzae* and *Strep. pneumoniae* are usually present in the sputum.

*Breathlessness* on effort first starts insidiously, but may be pro-minent on cold and foggy days. As the disease progresses, patients become more severely disabled with persistent breathlessness on exertion. The established bronchitic will usually have to stop at least once on one or two flights of stairs. Disabling breathlessness is the dominant feature preventing bronchitics from working. In the end stage of the disease the patient is breathless on even minimal exertion about the house, on getting into bed or dressing. Nocturnal breathlessness and cough often wake the patient from sleep, but this symptom may be missed unless a direct question is asked. Some believe that such nocturnal breathlessness indicates a measure of reversibility in the airways obstruction. Similar symptoms occur in the asthmatic, but here wheeze is usually dominant. Pulmonary oedema must also be considered as a cause of such 'paroxysmal nocturnal dyspnoea'.

*Haemoptysis* should never be regarded as a result of chronic bronchitis and emphysema alone, although it must be admitted that in some patients no other cause can be found. Bronchial carcinoma, tuberculosis or bronchiectasis should always be considered in a chronic bronchitic with haemoptysis. Chest pain is also unusual, unless pleurisy complicates a pneumonic episode. Some bronchitics are wheezy and it seems probable that persistent asthma, in which the airways obstruction is initially almost totally reversible, may eventually progress over the years to become irreversible, with exacerbations which may be indistinguishable clinically from established chronic bronchitis and emphysema.

# Physical signs

Relatively extensive emphysema is found at autopsy in over 60% of male smokers aged over 60 years, yet in most of these patients there will have been no indication of the disease during life. Early chronic bronchitis and emphysema may thus give rise to no physical signs. However, in the established disease *hyperinflation of the chest* is characteristic. This is shown by:

1. Indrawing of intercostal spaces and the supraclavicular fossa on inspiration, best detected in a good light by careful observation of the lower rib spaces. Although in a normal subject with a thin chest wall indrawing here may be seen on maximal inspiratory effort, intercostal indrawing over the pectoral region and in the supraclavicular fossa on quiet breathing is always pathological. The sign is seen on both sides and arises from the low intrapleural pressure generated by the inspiratory muscles, necessary to ventilate the hyperinflated (and therefore stiff) lungs through narrowed airways (see Chapter 1). This is easily verified in oneself by trying to take a normal breath on top of a previous large inspiration, which soon reveals the increased muscular effort that is needed.

2. Shortening of the distance between the cricoid cartilage and the suprasternal notch to less than three finger-breadths, which again can be quickly demonstrated on oneself, as this distance shortens as one breathes in.

3. Absence of the area of absolute cardiac dullness normally only found over the lower left quarter of the sternum (see Fig. 26).

4. Increase of the subcostal angle between the anterior margins of the two rib cages to over 90° (a less reliable sign).

5. An increase in the anteroposterior diameter of the chest may be present in hyperinflation, but this diameter is also increased in any condition which reduces the length of the thoracic spine, without at the same time reducing the volume of air in the chest. Thus kyphosis, osteoporosis with vertebral collapse and progressive reduction in the spinal length with advancing age, all tend to increase this diameter, so that it is a bad sign of hyperinflation of the chest.

Excessive use of the accessory muscles of respiration, particularly the sternomastoid muscles, is valuable if the patient does not know that he is being observed. Hyperresonance of the chest and decreased breath sounds are both *unreliable* signs of hyperinflation, for the disease affects both sides of the chest and thus the value of comparison between the two signs is lost. Coarse rhonchi, again throughout the chest, often predominantly at the bases, are a frequent sign indicating excess mucus secretion in large airways. In the hyperinflated chest heart sounds may be often best heard in the xiphisternal angle, and the apex beat if often difficult to locate.

Finger-clubbing is *not* found in simple chronic bronchitis and emphysema and must always lead to a search for other pathological processes, such as bronchial carcinoma, bronchiectasis etc.

*Central cyanosis* is best seen in the tongue in day light. It indicates deficiency of oxygenation of the arterial blood, with an arterial oxygen saturation below 90%, allthough occasionally it is difficult to detect until the saturation is below 85%. Simple arithmetic shows that the oft-quoted figure that the concentration of reduced haemoglobin is more than 5 g/dl when central cyanosis is detected, must mean that the saturation is then below 66%, if the patient has a normal haemoglobin concentration of 15 g/dl. At this level of arterial saturation (66%) the arterial $PO_2$ is dangerously low (4.67 kPa, 35 mmHg). This idea, although clearly indicating an incorrect concentration for the reduced haemoglobin (5 g/dl) is nonetheless correct in principle, for in fact a reduced haemoglobin concentration of 1.5–2 g/dl is detectable as central cyanosis. Thus in the polycythaemic patient cyanosis is easily recognized, but this is more difficult in the anaemic patient. Peripheral cyanosis is also present with central cyanosis, but the converse is not true. Central cyanosis in a patient breathing air at sea level indicates respiratory failure (see Chapter 11), as arterial hypoxaemia is present, if rare abnormal haemoglobin pigments (sulphaemoglobin and methaemoglobin) can be excluded. If this hypoxaemia is associated with a raised $PCO_2$ (Type II respiratory failure) the clinical signs *may* include a rapid pounding pulse, distended forearm veins and a flapping irregular tremor of the outstretched hands. However, all these signs may be absent in patients with a raised $PCO_2$, so that this can only be proved by arterial blood gas analysis. Engorgement of fundal veins is often found with a raised $PCO_2$, but papilloedema is rare.

### 'Pink and puffing' and 'blue and bloated'

Two patterns of chronic bronchitis and emphysema can be distinguished clinically, but most patients display some features of both patterns. The *'pink and puffing'* patient is characteristically thin, breathless, with marked hyperinflation of the chest, but without central cyanosis. Arterial blood gas analysis of this patient shows that he has a relatively normal $PO_2$ and $PCO_2$. Earlier ideas that this 'pink and puffing' pattern was predominantly associated with emphysema cannot be satisfactorily sustained by clinicopathological correlations.

The *'blue and bloated'* patient may not be particularly breathless, at least at rest, but has severe central cyanosis with signs of cor pulmonale (ankle oedema, occasionally ascites, an elevated jugular venous pressure and distended forearm veins). The arterial $PO_2$ is characteristically low, and the $PCO_2$ high (Type II respiratory failure) although the arterial pH is normal unless the patient is in an acute exacerbation (see Chapters 3 and 11). Earlier ideas that 'blue and bloated' patients had predominantly bronchitis with little emphysema are now also known to be in error. These patients can have much, some or almost no emphysema as shown by subsequent autopsy findings.

'Blue and bloated' patients are particularly prone to episodes of transient sleep hypoxaemia (Fig. 45) occurring recurrently throughout a normal night's sleep, when episodes of very low oxygen saturation occur in the rapid eye movement (REM) phase of sleep. The mechanism of these episodes of transient hypoxaemia is not yet fully established, but they are not due to a sleep apnoea syndrome alone (see Chapter 24), but occur more in episodes of transient hypoventilation.

The difference between the 'blue and bloated' and 'pink and puffing' patients with chronic bronchitis and emphysema is established on clinical grounds, but the underlying mechanism for these two patterns in patients with similar degrees of irreversible airways obstruction is still the subject of active research. One hypothesis suggests that the 'blue and bloated' are those who are born with a congenitally poor ventilatory response to hypoxia, whereas the 'pink

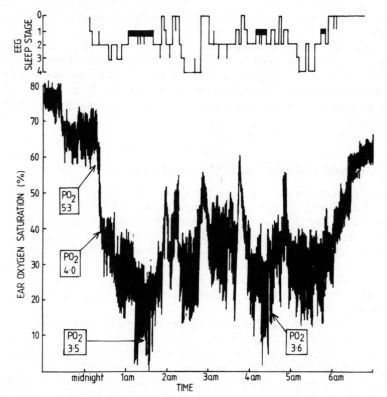

*Fig. 45.*   EEG sleep stage (o = drowsiness, 4 = deep sleep) and rapid eye movement ( ■, REM) sleep periods, above; arterial oxygen saturation (ear oximeter); and directly measured arterial $PO_2$ (kPa), throughout a night's sleep in a 'blue and bloated' patient with chronic bronchitis and emphysema, when breathing air

and puffing' have a particularly brisk response to this stimulus to breathing. This hypothesis, however, remains to be proved.

## Investigations

The *chest radiograph* may show hyperinflation of the chest, as shown by a flattened low diaphragm, revealing the eleventh rib in the postero-anterior view, with a long thin heart graphically described as the 'heart hung up to dry'. Earlier ideas that emphysema could be diagnosed accurately from the chest radiograph, particularly if there was a deficiency of peripheral vascular pattern in the lung fields, are now known to be erroneous. Even the world's best radiologist was only correct in his diagnosis of severe emphysema using such signs in 41% of cases later proved to have severe emphysema pathologically!

The characteristic radiographic appearance of the 'blue and bloated' patient with cor pulmonale will, of course, include an enlarged heart and prominent vascular shadows at both hila; in these patients hyperinflation, although present, is less obvious radiologically.

*Emphysematous bullae* may occur in any part of the lung fields, but are more common in the upper lobes. They appear as areas of hypertranslucency with absent pulmonary vascular markings, characteristically outlined by the hair-line shadow of the wall of the bulla.

*Respiratory function tests* are used to define the extent and severity of chronic bronchitis and emphysema and to indicate the response to treatment; *an obstructive pattern* with a low $FEV_1$, high TLC, an increased RV/TLC ratio, indicates hyperinflation. The ratio of $FEV_1$/FVC is usually below 70% but the FVC is also reduced as even a maximal expiratory effort will only partially deflate the lungs, due to the high residual volume (RV) (see Chapter 1). The transfer factor for carbon monoxide ($T$CO) is also below the predicted value for a patient of the same age, height and sex. This reduction in $T$CO, when coupled with the hyperinflation and low $FEV_1$, is the best functional indication of emphysema, but again extensive emphysema can exist with a relatively normal $T$CO.

*Arterial blood gas tension* measurements in the 'pink and puffing' patients show modest hypoxaemia when breathing air (arterial $PO_2$ 8–10 kPa; 60–75 mmHg), with a normal or low $PCO_2$, usually 4.7–6.0 kPa (35–45 mmHg), with a widening of the alveolar to arterial oxygen tension gradient (A–a$DO_2$) to 2.7–4.7 kPa (20–35 mmHg) and a normal arterial pH. In the 'blue and bloated', however, there is hypoxaemia, typical arterial $PO_2$ values when breathing air being 6.7–8.0 kPa (50–60 mmHg), with a similar $PCO_2$ and an A–a$DO_2$ around 4.7 kPa (35 mmHg). Again, the pH value will be normal in the chronic stable state.

In an *acute exacerbation*, when breathing air, hypoxaemia is often more profound, $PO_2$ values varying from 2.7 to 6.7 kPa (20–50 mmHg) with $PCO_2$ values between 6.7 and 12.0 kPa (50–90 mmHg), but higher values of $PCO_2$ are not encountered when these patients are breathing air, as this would mean that arterial $PO_2$ values would not be compatible with life. In addition, of course, the acute rise of $PCO_2$ in these patients due to hypoventilation implies acid–base values lying between the acute and chronic respiratory acidosis bands on the acid–base $[H^+]$/$PCO_2$ diagram (see Chapter 3). The severity of acidosis is a better guide to prognosis of an acute exacerbation than is the level of $PCO_2$ alone, for if the pH falls below 7.25 (or $[H^+]$ above 56 nmol/litre) during controlled oxygen therapy (see later) survival is less likely.

Other investigations show secondary polycythaemia with a high haemoglobin, red cell count, PCV and red cell mass in the 'blue and bloated'. Chronic carbon dioxide retention in these patients leads to a raised venous bicarbonate level due to an increased reabsorption of bicarbonate in the renal tubules, so compensating for the respiratory acidosis. Recent studies have suggested that secondary polycythaemia is particularly frequent in those patients who have chronically raised carboxyhaemoglobin levels (5–15%) from their persistent cigarette smoking.

## Cor pulmonale

Cor pulmonale can be defined clinically as right heart failure shown by ankle oedema, elevation of jugular venous pressure, and possibly hepatomegaly, due to chronic lung disease without pre-existing left ventricular failure. Pathologically the right ventricle is hypertrophied, as described earlier, and the mean pulmonary arterial pressure is raised, often to values between 25 and 50 mmHg at rest. This is part of the 'blue and bloated' pattern of chronic bronchitis and emphysema and the severity of both pulmonary hypertension and secondary polycythaemia relate to the severity of arterial hypoxaemia in these patients, when breathing air at rest in the chronic stable state. However, in the individual patient there is considerable variability in both responses. Other factors contribute to the pulmonary hypertension and secondary polycythaemia, as well as the hypoxaemia alone.

Right ventricular hypertrophy may be detected clinically by a sternal lift over the outflow tract of the right ventricle, but this is often obscured by the hyperinflated chest in these patients. However, the ECG shows right ventricular hypertrophy, with right axis deviation and dominance of the R wave in V4R, V3R and V1, possibly with inversion of T waves in the anterior chest leads. P pulmonale with P waves over 3 mm in height also indicates atrial hypertrophy, which is also characteristic of cor pulmonale in chronic bronchitis and emphysema (Fig. 46). The chest radiograph in these patients may show prominence of the hilar vascular shadows with bulging of the pulmonary artery conus to the left border of the cardiac outline (Fig. 47).

# Treatment

Treatment cannot restore functioning alveolar tissue which has been destroyed by emphysema, nor can it replace lost airways. However, the otherwise inexorable progression of the disease may be delayed by stopping smoking, improvement in airways obstruction and treatment of infective episodes. Rehabilitation procedures aim to enable the patient to make the most of his reduced respiratory reserve, so as to live a tolerable life within the limitations of his disease.

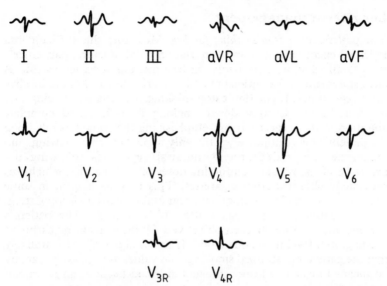

*Fig. 46.* Electrocardiogram in a 'blue bloater' with cor pulmonale and chronic bronchitis and emphysema, showing right ventricular hypertrophy, with P pulmonale, particularly well seen in lead 2

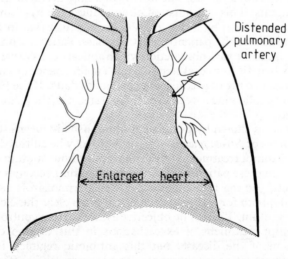

*Fig. 47.* Chest radiograph in a patient with cor pulmonale and pulmonary hypertension due to chronic bronchitis and emphysema

## Long-term management

The patient must *stop smoking for life*. Most find this difficult, but repeated encouragement and exhortation by all doctors, particularly their family doctor, is probably the best method of achieving this. A clear statement of the outlook must be given. 'Do you want to be alive in 10 years time?. If you don't stop smoking your chance of being so is much reduced'. Cutting down smoking is useless and complete abolition of the cigarette habit, emphasizing that this depends upon the patient's own willpower, is the only hope. Nicotine chewing gum (Nicorette) can reduce the withdrawal symptoms following deprivation of the regular reinforcing doses of the nicotine, which was previously obtained from cigarettes. This may be helpful in some patients. Anti-smoking clinics have regrettably proved disappointing, as most patients relapse again after initial success. The patient's perseverance can be checked objectively by measuring the carboxy-haemoglobin level in venous blood. If this is above 3%, it is unlikely that the patient has stopped smoking, and values as high as 15% are by no means unusual in heavy smokers in blood taken at an afternoon clinic.

*Airways obstruction* in these patients is relatively irreversible. However, even in severely disabled bronchitics with $FEV_1$ values around 0.5 litre, a combination of a *beta$_2$ sympathomimetic bronchodilator* (salbutamol, terbutaline, fenoterol) and the anti-cholinergic bronchodilator *ipratropium bromide*, both given as two puffs from a metered dose aerosol up to four times a day, can have a synergistic effect producing a modest but worthwhile improvement in $FEV_1$ in many patients. This combination often reduces the hyperinflation of the chest (as shown by a rise in FVC greater than that in $FEV_1$) so helping to relieve the patient's breathlessness. Patients with a history of wheeze, and airways obstruction which appears to have varied in the past, may benefit from oral steroids, but a maintenance dosage should never exceed 10 mg of prednisolone by mouth daily. If the $FEV_1$ does not improve following a week's trial of oral steroids, they should not be continued.

*Infection*, as shown by purulent sputum, usually means that either *H. influenzae* or *Strep. pneumoniae* (or both) may be cultured from the sputum. Prompt treatment with antibiotics without sputum culture is justifiable in these patients as soon as their sputum becomes purulent. Ampicillin, 500 mg four times a day, or co-trimoxazole two tablets twice daily, both for a 10-day course, can often clear these organisms from the sputum. There is no objective evidence from controlled trials that prompt treatment of exacerbations in this fashion can delay progression of the disease, but this antibiotic regimen is usually effective in clearing the sputum of pus and is certainly as effective, and much less expensive, than alternative regimens using cephalosporin antibiotics.

Infection with *influenza virus* (either A or B) can be very dangerous in these patients with severely compromised respiratory function. Prophylaxis by influenza vaccination should thus be given each October, the vaccine containing inactivated strains of the influenza virus currently recommended. Immunization against 14 of the most prevalent strains of *Strep. pneumoniae* is now available, using an inactivated vaccine. The efficacy of this has not yet been proved in patients with chronic bronchitis and emphysema, but it has been shown to prevent pneumonia from *Strep. pneumoniae* in other closed communities who are particularly at risk.

*Rehabilitation* aims to restore the fullest possible capability to these patients. Training of the respiratory muscles is currently under investigation, either using volume loading, with hyperventilation, or by breathing against a resistance. Early results suggest that these methods can improve exercise tolerance in patients with established chronic bronchitis and emphysema. Resistive loading can be carried out by the patient alone, using a facemask with a one-way valve and a series of tube connections to provide the requisite inspiratory resistance. This is carried out two or three times a day for 10–15 minutes. Exercise training has also been shown to improve the exercise tolerance of these patients, but as with all these techniques self-motivation by the patient is essential. Simple stair climbing can be used by the patient in his own home.

*Physiotherapy*, with teaching of 'breathing exercises' has been traditional, but nearly all attempts to assess the value of this treatment by objective measurements have either failed or produced conflicting results. Recent claims that an imposed breathing pattern with slow deep breathing, both at rest and during exercise, can improve exercise tolerance and reduce carbon dioxide retention and improve oxygenation have yet to be confirmed. Assisted coughing, possibly with postural drainage, can be of great value in clearing retained secretions in these patients.

*Long-term domiciliary oxygen therapy.* 'Blue and bloated' patients with hypoxic cor pulmonale have a grave prognosis. Two recent controlled trials have now shown that long-term oxygen therapy given at a flow rate of 2 litres of oxygen/minute by nasal prongs, over a period of 15 or more hours in the 24-hour day, can probably prolong the life of these patients (Fig. 48). The treatment is practicable, but expensive. It can be provided by oxygen cylinders delivered to the patient's home, 14 F size cylinders (48 ft$^3$, 1358 litres) being required each week. The cheapest supply is from the *oxygen concentrator*, a device the size of a domestic refrigerator which uses an electrical compressor to remove nitrogen from air, so yielding 90% or more oxygen. A liquid oxygen system (Union Carbide Walker, or Liberator/Stroller system) is intermediate in cost between cylinders and the concentrator, but can provide oxygen therapy on exercise for the mobile patient. However, these liquid systems require a delivery of liquid oxygen twice per week to the patient's home. Nocturnal oxygen therapy, to prevent the development of pulmonary hypertension during the transient sleep hypoxaemia of the 'blue and bloated' bronchitic, has yet to be established. American studies have suggested that survival with continuous oxygen therapy in such patients is better than that with nocturnal oxygen therapy alone. Exacerbation of acute chronic $CO_2$ retention by this controlled oxygen therapy does not seem to be a major problem in these patients. Smoking during oxygen therapy is very dangerous. Provision of long-term oxygen therapy for the patient with a persistently raised carboxyhaemoglobin level from smoking is probably not justifiable.

## Treatment of an acute exacerbation

Acute exacerbations, with increased severity of hypoxaemia and carbon dioxide retention with respiratory acidosis, can be precipitated by influenza or infection with *Strep. pneumoniae* and *Haemophilus influenzae*. In a severe influenza epidemic, staphylococcal pneumonia is an ever-present threat to these patients. Development of a pneumothorax, trivial trauma causing a fractured rib, or injudicious use of hypnotics or narcotic analgesics (nitrazepam, barbiturates, morphine etc.) are all recognized as precipitants of an acute exacerbation in these patients. Such a patient will characteristically be centrally cyanosed and drowsy but not usually complaining of severe breathlessness. Diagnosis of such an exacerbation with Type II respiratory failure (hypoxaemia and carbon dioxide retention; see Chapter 11) depends upon recognizing the possibility in such a cyanosed patient, the diagnosis then being confirmed by measurement of arterial blood gas tensions. The physical signs of carbon dioxide retention (rapid bounding pulse, warm skin, distended forearm veins, irregular flapping tremor of the outstretched hands, headache, drowsiness and coma) can all be fallacious, as they may be caused by many other conditions, and indeed may be absent in patients with life-threatening carbon dioxide retention and respiratory acidosis.

### Controlled oxygen therapy

These patients are in danger of death from hypoxaemia. However, relief of this hypoxaemia by injudicious high concentrations of oxygen can thereby remove a stimulus to breathing, so allowing carbon dioxide retention to become more severe, so that the patient dies in respiratory acidosis. This is known as carbon dioxide narcosis. This sequence can be avoided by *controlled oxygen therapy*, which aims to provide enough oxygen to prevent death from hypoxaemia without precipitating severe respiratory acidosis. This is achieved in the first instance by 2 litres/minute of oxygen by nasal prongs, or alternatively by a 28% Ventimask, or Edinburgh mask at 2 litres/minute, following the initial diagnostic arterial blood gas estimation. This is repeated one hour after starting controlled oxygen, to ensure that the arterial $PO_2$ is over 6.7 kPa (50 mmHg), without the arterial pH having fallen below 7.25 ([$H^+$] over 56 nmol/litre). The severity of the acidosis is a better guide to prognosis in these patients than is the $PCO_2$ value for many suffer from acute-on-chronic carbon dioxide retention.

If the above limits cannot be achieved, the respiratory stimulant drug doxapram is given by continuous intravenous infusion, in a dose ranging from 0.5 mg/minute to 4.0 mg/minute, using a concentration of 2 mg/ml in 5% dextrose. The dosage is titrated to provide the desired arterial blood gas tensions and pH ($PO_2$ over 6.7 kPa (50 mmHg), pH over 7.25 and [$H^+$] under 56 nmol/litre), while controlled oxygen therapy is continued. The side effects of doxapram include tremor, tachycardia, burning pain in the perineum, and agitation, but the drug is undoubtedly a powerful analeptic. If, despite this regimen, the stated limits of $PO_2$ and [$H^+$] cannot be achieved, consideration should be given to the institution of mechanical ventilation by a cuffed endotracheal tube. However, many of these patients have repeated acute exacerbations and the possibility of restoring a worthwhile existence must be carefully considered before this expensive and distressing treatment is started. Mechanical ventilation using intermittent positive pressure in these patients is difficult, as the high airways resistance and hyperinflation (low compliance) means that high inflation pressures are required, so tending to impede the venous return and reduce the cardiac output. Ventilation should therefore be adjusted to obtain a normal arterial pH (or [$H^+$]) and *not* an arbitrary normal $PCO_2$ value, for this latter can cause severe respiratory alkalosis due to the chronic bicarbonate retention which these patients have maintained over many years. Controlled oxygen therapy, doxapram infusion, and mechanical ventilation all attempt to control the respiratory failure and thus maintain life, whilst the cause of the exacerbation of chronic bronchitis and emphysema is being treated.

*Treatment of the cause of respiratory failure* will depend upon finding what this is. In most patients an exacerbation of bronchial infection causes the problem, with or without bronchopneumonia. Ampicillin or co-trimoxazole (as discussed above) are efficient agents for treating *H. influenzae* or *Strep. pneumoniae* infections, but in an influenza epidemic or the desperately ill patient it is wise to assume that a staphylococcal infection may be present (see Staphylococcal pneumonia; Chapter 8). When sputum culture results are available chemotherapy may be later adjusted. A chest radiograph serves to exclude a pneumothorax, which unless trivial should always be treated with intercostal under-water sealed drain in these patients; or a fractured rib causing pleuritic pain can prevent adequate ventilation of the adjacent alveoli. An intercostal nerve block can be used to relieve

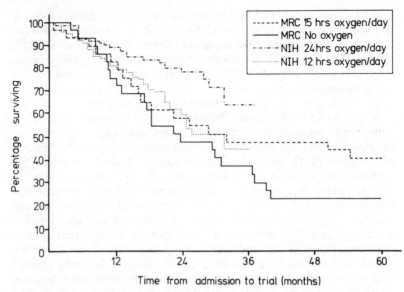

*Fig. 48.*    Survival of 'blue and bloated' patients with chronic bronchitis
and emphysema treated without long-term oxygen and with
various long-term oxygen regimens in two recent British (MRC)
and American (NIH) trials

this vicious cycle, as adequate analgesia with narcotics is
contraindicated as a result of their respiratory depressant action.
Injudicious use of such narcotics can precipitate respiratory failure,
which may be reversed by naloxone 0.4 mg intravenously or intramuscularly. Pulmonary oedema from a myocardial infarction can
cause respiratory failure in these patients, but usually responds to
diuretics.

## Prognosis

The outlook for the patient with established chronic bronchitis and
emphysema, particularly if this has progressed to the 'blue and
bloated' pattern with cor pulmonale, pulmonary hypertension, secondary polycythaemia and persistent Type II respiratory failure, is very
grave (Fig. 48). Thus in a recent study of 111 such patients who left
hospital following an acute exacerbation, only 30% were alive five
years later.

## Further reading

BATES, D. V., MACKLEM, P. T. and CHRISTIE, R. V. (1971) *Respiratory Function
in Disease*, 2nd ed. Philadelphia: W. B. Saunders.

FLENLEY, D. C. and WARREN, P. M. (1980) Chronic bronchitis and emphysema. In *Recent Advances in Respiratory Medicine II*, ed. D. C. Flenley. Edinburgh: Churchill Livingstone.

MRC WORKING PARTY (1981) Long term domiciliary oxygen therapy in hypoxic cor pulmonale complicating chronic bronchitis and emphysema. *Lancet, 1*, 681–685.

MAY, J. R. (1972) *The Chemotherapy of Chronic Bronchitis and Allied Disorders*, 2nd ed. London: English University Press.

ROYAL COLLEGE OF PHYSICIANS (1981) Disabling chest disease: prevention and care. *J. R. Coll. Physcns*, **15**, 3.

THURLBECK, W. M. (1976) *Major Problems in Pathology, V. Chronic Airflow Obstruction in Lung Disease*. Philadelphia: W. B. Saunders.

WOOLCOCK, A. J. (1980) The pathogenesis of chronic obstructive lung disease with particular reference to the small airway hypothesis. In *Recent Advances in Respiratory Medicine II*, ed. D. C. Flenley. Edinburgh: Churchill Livingstone.

# 10

# Bronchial Asthma

Bronchial asthma is characterized by recurrent episodes of acute limitation of air flow, remitting either spontaneously or in response to treatment.

## Epidemiology

The disease can occur for the first time at any age, but is commoner in children, where it may afflict up to 4% of the childhood population in Europe, and possibly more in Japan and America; it is by no means unknown in the tropics where it is characteristically found in urban communities. In childhood boys are about twice as often affected as girls. Many children improve later in childhood, the disease often remitting more or less completely around puberty. Asthma starting in adults probably occurs in about 1% of the population, but it is being recognized increasingly often in older people.

## Types of asthma

Two types of asthma are recognized: the first, the *atopic* (extrinsic), is distinguished by clear recognition of an allergic precipitating factor, which in Britain is often the house dust mite (*Dermatophagoides pteronynissinus*) or grass pollens and in the USA often ragweed pollen. In these patients the condition usually starts in childhood, there is usually a family history of asthma or hay fever in one or more blood relatives, the child has often had eczema in infancy, and rarely this may persist into adult life (the asthma/eczema syndrome) with chronic eczema (Besnier's prurigo). The second type, much less frequent in childhood, but of equal incidence to atopic asthma when the condition starts in the adult, is *non-atopic* (intrinsic) where a causal allergen cannot be identified. These patients rarely have a family history of asthma, no hay fever, eczema or other allergic manifestations. Their attacks are not related to the seasonal incidence of pollens, as for example grass pollens in summer.

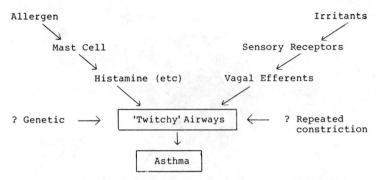

*Fig. 49.*   Precipitation of an attack of asthma, by interaction of a trigger (irritant or allergen) with hyperactive or 'twitchy' airways

# Aetiology and pathogenesis

Two factors seem essential to precipitate an attack of asthma (Fig. 49):

1. *Bronchial hyper-reactivity* describes the excessive increase in airways resistance which follows non-allergic challenge of the asthmatic by inhalation of histamine, prostaglandin $F_{2\alpha}$, sulphur dioxide or dust particles, all of which produce bronchoconstriction at concentrations much lower than that necessary to produce the same degree of airways resistance in a normal subject. These responses are often blocked by atropine, suggesting that vagal efferent nerves contribute to this bronchoconstriction.

2. *Allergic bronchial constriction* is characteristically shown as a Type I immune reaction, dependent upon an increase in specific circulating IgE (reagin) resulting from an immune response to previous exposure to the allergen. Specific circulating IgE can be detected by the radioallergosorbent test (RAST), but as this correlates well with the reaction to skin prick tests, these expensive RAST tests are rarely carried out in clinical practice. The allergen molecule binds two dimers of IgE to the receptors of those mast cells probably lying superficial to the basement membrane of the airways, and this causes the mast cell to release preformed mediators of anaphylaxis: histamine, eosinophil chemotactic factor (ECF-A), neutrophil chemotactic factor (NCF-A) and the unstored mediators, notably the slow-reacting substance of anaphylaxis (SRS-A) (now synthesized as a lipoxygenation product of arachidonic acid) and platelet activating factor (PAF) (Fig. 50). These substances are then thought to increase the permeability of the basement membrane of the airways, so allowing further molecules of allergen to penetrate and so interact with IgE molecules on the surface of the majority of the mast cells, which lie

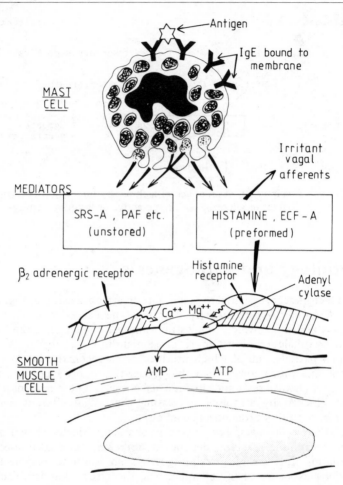

*Fig. 50.*    Summary of some of the factors involved in antigen-mediated bronchoconstriction. Antigen binding to two IgE molecules on the mast cell membrane releases mediators, which in turn act on receptor sites on the smooth muscle cells to change intracellular cyclic AMP levels, so promoting muscular contraction

deep to this membrane. The mediators act on bronchial smooth muscle, via the adenyl cyclase in the wall of the muscle cells, to decrease intracellular cyclic AMP concentrations, which thus promotes muscular contraction. This results in bronchoconstriction and the asthmatic attack.

**Familial factors**

Despite much research the genetic predisposition to atopic asthma remains obscure and is undoubtedly complex. Circulating levels of IgE are genetically determined in man. Thus, for example, the average level of IgE is some three times higher in Filipino–American children than in Caucasian children, and the incidence of atopic disease was higher in the Filipinos. Furthermore, the IgE response to specific antigens in unrelated allergic patients is associated with certain specific histocompatibility (HLA) genes. The immune response (Ir) genes which determine such responses in both animals and man are closely associated in the genome with this HLA gene complex. Nonetheless, the HLA phenotype does not relate to the prevalence of atopic asthma in patients.

# Pathology

Death in asthma is rare, usually unexpected and often occurs at night. At autopsy the airways are plugged with mucus, the bronchial walls show hyperplasia of mucous glands and of bronchial smooth muscle, with a submucosal inflammatory reaction with dilated capillaries and interstitial oedema, and the bronchi are infiltrated with eosinophils. Oedema can cause the mucous membrane to be shed completely and exfoliated ciliary epithelial cells are then found in the mucus plugs.

Mucosal oedema, hyperaemia and airway narrowing have been directly observed in the bronchi of atopic asthmatics within 10 minutes of instilling antigen onto the bronchial mucosa, as this process was watched through a fibreoptic bronchoscope.

# Functional disturbances

The bronchoconstriction of an asthmatic attack is easily shown by repeated measurements of $FEV_1$, FVC or peak flow following inhalation of an antigen in an atopic asthmatic, a technique known as bronchial challenge (Fig. 51). These tests can be dangerous, are not indicated in routine assessment and should only be performed with careful clinical supervision, with bronchodilators and steroids being available. Rarely a delayed or *late reaction* occurs some six to eight hours after the initial challenge (Fig. 51). This is usually thought to indicate a Type III immune reaction, caused by interaction of IgE antigen within the bronchial tissues, activating complement and subsequent release of anaphylotoxins. This late reaction can be blocked by steroids and also usually by sodium cromoglycate, which would argue against such a late reaction being a Type III response.

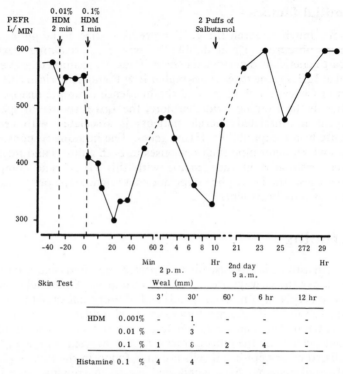

*Fig. 51.*   Serial measurements of peak expiratory flow (PEF) following bronchial challenge by inhalation of a diluted house mite extract in an atopic asthmatic who has skin hypersensitivity to the extract. Note the immediate and delayed responses

Similar late bronchoconstriction can occur following small molecular weight chemicals which are known to cause occupational asthma, i.e. the complex salts of platinum, soldering flux and toluene di-isocyanate, although precipitating antibodies to these substances cannot be demonstrated.

# Clinical features

The *acute attack* usually occurs spontaneously, but with hindsight may be related to bronchial infection or allergen exposure. Breathlessness and wheeze are the major complaints, with a 'tightness' in the chest, which must not be confused with angina. Cough may initiate the attack, but sputum production is rare and breathlessness becomes the dominant feature, with the patient sitting forward gasping for breath.

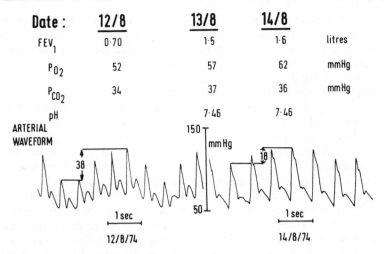

| Date : | 12/8 | 13/8 | 14/8 | |
|---|---|---|---|---|
| FEV$_1$ | 0·70 | 1·5 | 1·6 | litres |
| P$_{O_2}$ | 52 | 57 | 62 | mmHg |
| P$_{CO_2}$ | 34 | 37 | 36 | mmHg |
| pH | | 7·46 | 7·46 | |

*Fig. 52.*  Pulsus paradoxus in an acute attack of asthma with a low FEV$_1$, hypoxaemia and low $P_{CO_2}$, gradually improving, when FEV$_1$ was almost doubled to 1.6 litres, but hypoxaemia persisted ($P_{O_2}$ 62 mmHg), although pulsus paradoxus was much reduced

Examination reveals the obvious respiratory distress, indrawing of the supraclavicular fossae and intercostal spaces, and sometimes hyperinflation with shortening of cricosternal distance, with diminution of the area of absolute cardiac dullness. Wheeze is often audible without the stethoscope, but with it high-pitched rhonchi throughout the lung fields are characteristic. A severe attack is indicated by the patient's inability to speak, central cyanosis (which may be difficult to recognize due to the vasoconstriction associated with a low $P_{CO_2}$ characteristic of the asthmatic attack), tachycardia (pulse rate over 120/minute in the adult) and pulsus paradoxus (see Fig. 52), where the peripheral pulses may appear to vanish entirely on inspiration. A patient showing such signs *needs urgent treatment*.

As in any intermittent illness, the diagnosis must often be made from the patient's account (or that of his relatives) or other eye witnesses. The patient may be normal between attacks. Without treatment attacks can last 12–48 hours, but minor attacks may only last for an hour or two, and often characteristically *wake the patient from sleep* in the early hours, but this symptom is often only revealed by a direct question. Wheeze is frequently worse first thing in the morning. This pattern of nocturnal wheeze has been described as the 'morning dip' pattern, from the fall in FEV$_1$ or peak flow which is then demonstrable, and proper enquiry shows that it is unusual for an atopic asthmatic never to have had such nocturnal or early morning wheeze. Attacks which occur only in the summer, often preceded by hay fever (watering and itching of the eyes, sneezing and possibly watery nasal discharge) are common in asthma due to grass pollen allergy. Conversely, perennial asthma may be worse in the winter months, starting in the autumn, and is commonly found to be due to house mite sensitivity, at least in northern Europe.

*Exercise-induced asthma*, where wheeze follows running, is very common in children with atopic asthma, but again can only be revealed usually on direct questioning, such as 'What happens when you run for a bus?' and 'What happens during the run, after catching the bus, and then sitting down?'. These questions may reveal the characteristic answer of wheeze and tightness in the chest after the exertion.

*Late-onset asthma* may be a recurrence of early childhood asthma, which at first is forgotten. It may well be atopic, as shown by positive skin prick tests (see later), but in many of these patients no allergen can be demonstrated. *Allergic bronchopulmonary aspergillosis* is always a diagnostic possibility in a patient with late-onset asthma, and may be indicated by persistence of the wheeze despite treatment, by eosino-philia in both blood and sputum (see Chapter 24), transient opacities on the chest radiograph, possibly with 'tram-lining' and ring shadows due to thickening of bronchial walls, and aspergillin pre-cipitins present in the serum. Hyphae of the fungus are sometimes found in the sputum, but are not essential for the diagnosis, and it is more common for the fungus to be cultured from the sputum in such cases. Hyphae are nearly always present in a mucus plug which may be coughed up as a bronchial cast in the sputum in bronchopulmonary aspergillosis.

*Aspirin* is recognized as provoking asthma in possibly 1–10% of asthmatics. These patients classically develop an intermittent watery nasal discharge in their thirties, followed by recurrent nasal polyps. Asthma then develops in the next few years, the attack following oral aspirin, although this could previously be taken with impunity. There is no sensitivity to other common allergens, but other analgesics (e.g. indomethacin, ibuprofen, phenylbutazone and paracetamol) can pro-voke attacks, as can the yellow–orange dyestuff tartrazine, which is often present in foodstuffs and soft drinks. Inhibition of prostaglandin synthetase by these agents may lead to release of SRS-A, which causes the bronchospasm. Avoidance of these drugs, or tartrazine, prevents attacks.

# Investigations

The essential feature of asthma is airways obstruction, which may be shown by a reduction in peak expiratory flow (PEF), and $FEV_1$ or $FEV_1/FVC$ ratio. All these measurements may be normal between attacks, although in the patient with persistent recurrent attacks of asthma from childhood, persistent airways obstruction begins to develop after several years, and this is less readily completely reversible by standard bronchodilators. The asthmatic in an attack shows the classical obstructive pattern of respiratory function, the low $FEV_1/FVC$ ratio being associated with hyperinflation and very large total lung capacity. However, such measurements are rarely carried out as these patients will not tolerate breathing into respiratory apparatus during an attack. Blood gas abnormalities are usual during a severe attack of asthma, hypoxaemia breathing air being associated with a *low* $PCO_2$ and *respiratory alkalosis*. A *rise in* $PCO_2$ in an asthmatic is a very serious sign and is an indication for urgent consideration of the need for mechanical ventilation. Hypoxaemia results from ventilation/perfusion imbalance and may persist for several days with $PO_2$ values when breathing air as low as 5.3 kPa (40 mmHg) not being unusual in an acute attack. Blood and sputum eosinophilia is characteristic of allergic asthma and the raised IgE levels correlate well with skin sensitivity to common allergens. The chest radiograph is usually normal in asthma, but spontaneous pneumothorax is always a danger in the acute asthmatic attack, and may be clinically very difficult to detect in such patients. The 'silent chest', where the wheeze appears to vanish, is the hallmark of very severe status asthmaticus. Chest radiograph in these patients is mandatory, particularly if mechanical ventilation is to be commenced, for they can be killed by cardiac tamponade if a pneumothorax is not relieved urgently.

*Skin prick tests* are commonly used to detect specific circulating IgE After cleaning the anterior surface of the forearm with soap and water only, a drop of the control and allergen solutions to be tested are placed on the skin, and then pricked just into the dermis without drawing blood, using a fine needle. After 10–20 minutes the reactions are read by noting the diameter of any weal, in comparison to that to the control solution. A reaction of 10 mm diameter is strongly positive, 3 mm less so, etc. The common inhaled allergens are most reliable, including extract of the house mite, grass pollens, feathers, animal furs, etc. Corticosteroids do not interfere with this Type I immune response, but it is possible that antihistamines or sympathomimetics may do so.

# Treatment

Treatment is best considered as that of the acute attack of asthma, followed by preventive treatment which aims to inhibit the development of further attacks of asthma.

# The acute attack

Treatment of the acute attack is a crescendo of therapeutic endeavour. The patient with asthma will usually start treatment of an attack himself, by use of the inhaler of sympathomimetic bronchodilators (salbutamol or terbutaline), of which two puffs may be taken every four hours. If this self-medication does not work, further assistance will usually be sought. The *severe attack* requiring hospital admission and urgent treatment is recognized by central cyanosis, inability to speak sentences, tachycardia with a pulse rate over 120/minute in the adult, and marked pulsus paradoxus. Such patients need oxygen at a flow rate of at least 2 litres/minute by nasal prongs, but higher concentrations carry no danger as the $PCO_2$ is usually low. When oxygen is being given, intravenous aminophylline, in a dose of 500 mg slowly over five minutes by intravenous injection, can be given, followed by intravenous hydrocortisone in a dose of 150 mg. Assisted ventilation through a mouthpiece or mask with a pressure cycled ventilator (Bennett or Bird) can be used to deliver salbutamol or terbutaline directly to the airways, using the ventilator solution nebulized by this mechanical ventilator. Using the Bird respirator nebulized terbutaline (as the respirator solution) containing 10 mg/ml can be used, 5 mg being given in most cases, the total dose not exceeding 10 mg. Salbutamol as a respirator solution is diluted to 50–100 $\mu$g/ml, the total dose of salbutamol being 1–2 mg per hour.

Serum potassium levels should be measured in the acute asthmatic, for both corticosteroids and $\beta_2$ sympathomimetics can cause serious hypokalaemia.

These measures will usually relieve the severe asthmatic attack within six to 24 hours, but repeated intravenous aminophylline and hydrocortisone may be needed, to a total dose of 1000 mg of hydrocortisone in the first 24 hours. Oxygen should be continued for at least 48–72 hours following a severe attack of asthma, and it is advisable for the patient to remain in bed until the pulse rate is persistently below 100/minute. Oral steroid therapy, with 60 mg prednisolone in the 24-hour day, should also start as soon as the patient can swallow satisfactorily, and then continue in reducing dosage to 60 mg a day for two days, 40 mg a day for two days, reducing by 10 mg per two days, and later by 5 mg every second day, to a daily maintenance dose of not more than 10 mg within one week or so of the severe attack. Again as the patient improves aerosol bronchodilator therapy, with salbutamol or terbutaline by metered dose aerosol, can be substituted for wet nebulized bronchodilators delivered by intermittent positive pressure breathing using the respirator solutions.

## Preventing recurrent attacks

The mainstay here is aerosol medication, regular beclomethasone metered aerosol steroid being given as two puffs three or four times daily. This is particularly valuable for the atopic asthmatic and may be combined with salbutamol, terbutaline or fenoterol by metered dose aerosol, given as two puffs which are taken not more often than every four hours. This regimen is also used for early initial treatment of any attack of asthma that may occur. It should be emphasized to the patient that the beclomethasone is intended to prevent the attacks and so must be taken regularly, whether they feel wheezy or not. In asthmatics over 40 years of age, there is some advantage in combining this with ipratropium bromide, an atropine-like drug which inhibits vagally mediated bronchoconstriction. This is taken by metered dose inhaler, two puffs three or four times a day, and can follow the beclomethasone inhalation.

Patients should be instructed in the correct way to use aerosol therapy. Following one or two complete breaths, after full expiration, the metered dose inhaler is placed between the lips, and during a rapid inspiration the cannister is depressed so as to release one puff of the aerosol into the inspiratory gas flow. The patient should then hold his breath for a few seconds at full inspiration and then breath out slowly. Terbutaline is now available with a 'spacer' added to the aerosol inhaler, which appears to assist even distribution of the aerosol within the respiratory tract and so is particularly useful for patients who have difficulty in coordinating the inhaling movement. The patient's use of any metered dose aerosol should be checked.

*Oral theophyllines*, particularly proprietary preparations designed to improve absorption from the gastrointestinal tract, have been helpful in some patients and are widely used in North America, where metered dose aerosols of modern $\beta_2$ sympathomimetics are not widely available. For maximal effect, theophylline should be given to reach a serum level of 5–15 $\mu$g/ml, higher levels giving toxic effects, including tremor, tachycardia and eventually serious ventricular arrhythmias and epileptic fits if very high doses are given. Nausea and gastrointestinal discomfort are common, however, with many oral preparations of theophylline. Slow-release oral salbutamol, 4–8 mg by mouth, may help to relieve wheeze at night, which is now recognized to be a very frequent symptom in the asthmatic.

*Disodium cromoglycate* stabilizes the mast cell against degranulation and was a valuable addition to therapy for asthma. The drug is taken by inhalation as a powder from a 'spinhaler', in a dose of one capsule, taken not more often than four times daily. Cromoglycate is particularly valuable in patients with a clear history of exercise-induced asthma and, if taken two to four hours before the exercise, can often prevent the development of this distressing symptom. The drug has no side effects.

A recent innovation has been an anti-allergic drug with sedative and antihistaminic properties, *ketotifen*, which is active orally. The drug causes drowsiness early in the course of treatment and its role as a substitute for inhaled cromoglycate is still being evaluated.

## Drug interactions in asthma

Drugs interacting with the action of sympathomimetic amines can precipitate an asthmatic attack and render treatment difficult. Beta blockers (propranolol, metoprolol, oxprenolol, etc.) can all have this effect, and such drugs are probably contraindicated in the proved asthmatic (see Chapter 21). Antihistamines have no action in asthma and this also applies to cimetidine (the $H_2$ blocker) which is not contraindicated in the asthmatic.

## Practical management of asthma

Many patients are children or young adults and the history will often give a clear guide to the presence of atopy, which can be confirmed by skin tests, which in the UK will often reveal positive reactions to house mite or grass pollens. The avoidance of such allergens is rarely completely practical and simple measures such as damp dusting, removal of dust traps in the child's bedroom and confining dust-raising activity to the morning when the child is out are all reasonable, but most physicians feel that encasing the mattress in a plastic bag is scarcely worthwhile. The house mite is relatively ubiquitous in northern Europe, and also in tropical Africa, and total avoidance is impractical. Desensitization to house mite has not been shown by controlled trials to be of value. Drug therapy, starting with sympathomimetic inhaled metered dose aerosols (salbutamol, terbutaline, fenoterol, etc.) can be combined with sodium cromoglycate if exercise-induced asthma is a major problem. Strongly positive skin tests suggest that beclomethasone combined with the sympathomimetic bronchodilators may be helpful. If these measures do not succeed in preventing recurrent attacks of asthma, oral steroids, in a maintenance dose for the adult of not exceeding 10 mg prednisolone per day, can be employed. In children and adolescents steroids can inhibit growth and there is marginal advantage in preventing this by using intramuscular tetracosactrin, two or three times per week by intramuscular injection. In children of school age a maintenance dose of 0.25–1 mg tetracosactrin two or three times a week may be required to control symptoms. Intermittent higher doses of intermittent oral steroids may avoid the need for such injections, with only a minor risk of inhibiting growth from premature fusion of epiphyses, but the exact doses and duration of courses will have to depend upon the individual patient's condition.

The severe asthmatic should preferably be listed on an *emergency admission register*, held at a hospital, and allowed to arrange self-admission to the hospital, equipped to treat the acute attack of asthma, without the necessity for referral to a general practitioner. Some patients may benefit from wet nebulization (pressure-driven nebulizer) at home using either salbutamol or terbutaline respirator solutions in place of the metered dose aerosol, and this has been successfully used in treating children with severe asthma at home. The intelligent adult can be advised to treat a bad attack of asthma, which has not responded to metered dose of sympathomimetics by inhalation, by using oral steroids. A dose of 30 mg of prednisolone is taken on the first day, followed by reduction of one 5 mg tablet on each of the next days, to cease the drug altogether within six days. This regimen can be used without medical supervision, but should not be used more often than once a month, with the general rule that a prolonged dose of prednisolone of more than 10 mg/day should be avoided.

Most children with asthma outgrow their disease at around puberty, but this is less likely in those who have had severe persistent attacks in childhood, and such patients may become permanently dependent on maintenance steroid therapy, but nonetheless acute exacerbations of asthma punctuate the course of their illness. Death in asthma is rare, but usually occurs unexpectedly and not infrequently following discharge from hospital after the apparently successful treatment of an acute attack, and then often at night. Many believe that any asthmatic who survives to be admitted to hospital should very rarely die, but asthma still causes 1000 to 2000 deaths each year in the United Kingdom. The suspicion remains that efficient delivery of our present methods of treatment should reduce this figure, this idea lying behind the emergency asthma self-admission schemes available for known severe asthmatics.

Asthma starting in adult life is often non-atopic and is usually more difficult to treat, with a consequently worse prognosis. It seems probable that chronic persistent asthma eventually progresses to a stage of relatively irreversible airways obstruction, such patients then having very similar clinical features to the patient with established chronic bronchitis and emphysema. However, such patients can be recognized by careful history taking, but at this stage in the progressive persistent disease, bronchodilatation with sympathomimetics, anticholinergic agents and steroids may still fail to restore normal airway calibre. Asthma in patients with bronchopulmonary aspergillosis is often severe and may only be controlled with unacceptable high doses of oral steroids. Atopic asthma can occur in the elderly and can respond satisfactorily to simple treatment with steroids and sympathomimetic aerosols.

*Side effects of prolonged high dosage steroid therapy* result both from the inhibition of the normal pituitary adrenal axis, so that stress (infection, trauma, etc.) does not lead to the normal increase in output of endogenous adrenal steroids, and from the direct pharmacological actions of the steroids themselves. Any patient on long-term steroids should be warned to tell his doctors that he is on such treatment if he requires surgery for accidents, etc., for the dose may need to be temporarily increased, as also for the stress of a serious inter-current infection. Pharmacological side effects include mooning of the face, obesity of the trunk, purple striae of the skin of the abdomen, buttocks and shoulders, hypertension, osteoporosis, induction of diabetes mellitus, psychosis, hypokalaemic alkalosis and susceptibility to infection; thus it is necessary to keep the dose as low as possible to control the disease. These effects are all very rare if a dose of 10 mg/day is not exceeded in the adult. Nonetheless, patients receiving such long-term steroid therapy are best supervised by three- or six-monthly checks on body weight, blood pressure and presence of sugar in the urine. Enquiry should then be directed to back pain or change of mood. A child born to an asthmatic mother who has received steroids during pregnancy may require steroids followed by ACTH if vomiting or a rising serum potassium indicates adrenal failure.

## Further reading

BOUSHEY, H. A., HOLTZMAN, M. J., SHELLER, J. R. and NADEL, J. A. (1980) Bronchial hyperreactivity. *Am. Rev. resp. Dis.*, **121**, 389–413.

CLARK, T. J. H. and GODFREY, S. (1977) *Asthma*. London: Chapman and Hall.

DANIEL, H. D. and SCHROMM, K. (1980) New pharmaceutical agents for the treatment of bronchial asthma. In *Recent Advances in Respiratory Medicine II*, ed. D. C. Flenley. Edinburgh: Churchill Livingstone.

LEADER (1980) Aspirin sensitivity in asthma. *Br. med. J.*, **2**, 958–959.

LICHTENSTEIN, L. M. and AUSTEN, K. F. (1977) *Asthma; Physiology, Immunopharmacology and Treatment*. New York: Academic Press.

MARSH, D. G., HSU, S. H., HUSSAIN, R. et al. (1980) Genetics of human immune response to allergens. *J. Allergy clin. Immunol.*, **65**, 322–332.

NADEL, J. A. (1980) *Lung Biology in Health and Disease, 15. Physiology and Pharmacology of the Airways*. New York and Basel: Marcel Dekker.

PORTER, R. and BIRCH, J. (1971) *Identification of Asthma. Ciba Foundation Study Group, No. 38*, Edinburgh: Churchill Livingstone.

# Respiratory Failure and the Adult Respiratory Distress Syndrome

## Respiratory failure

The respiratory function of the lungs is gas exchange, so that respiratory failure is defined in terms of gas tensions of blood leaving the lungs — the arterial $PO_2$, $PCO_2$ and pH. Respiratory failure is present in a patient breathing air at sea level if the arterial $PO_2$ is less than 8.0 kPa (60 mmHg), as a result of lung disease. If this arterial $PO_2$ is combined with a normal or low $PCO_2$ (below 6.7 kPa, 50 mmHg), this is *type I respiratory failure*; if in addition to the hypoxaemia the $PCO_2$ is raised (above 6.7 kPa, 500 mmHg), *type II respiratory failure* is present.

### Type I respiratory failure

*Causes*

Type I respiratory failure (low $PO_2$, low or normal $PCO_2$) arises most frequently from an increased variability in ventilation/perfusion ratios between the different alveoli of the lungs. As a result of the differing shapes of the oxygen and carbon dioxide dissociation curves of blood, hyperventilation of some alveoli with a normal blood flow (thus a high $\dot{V}a/\dot{Q}$) cannot compensate by adding sufficient extra oxygen to the blood stream from that oxygen deficiency resulting from under-ventilation of other alveoli with a normal blood supply (low $\dot{V}a/\dot{Q}$). Thus, the arterial blood leaving such a mixture of alveoli will have a lower than normal $PO_2$, in comparison with that if both sets of alveoli had a normal ventilation and blood flow. In contrast, however, as the carbon dioxide dissociation curve is almost linear in the physiological range, hyperventilation of some alveoli can compensate for hypoventilation of other alveoli, in terms of $PCO_2$ (Fig. 53).

A less common, but well recognized, cause of type I respiratory failure is an increase in perfusion of alveoli which effectively receive no blood supply, so forming a 'shunt' or admixture of venous blood directly to the arterial blood leaving the lungs, so causing a fall in arterial $PO_2$. Here, increase in inspired oxygen concentration will have

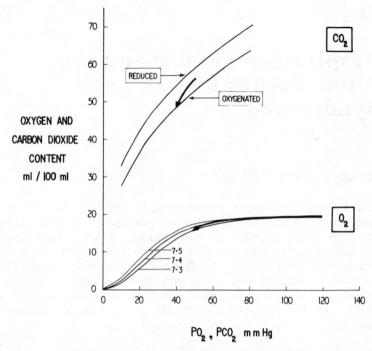

*Fig. 53.*   Oxygen and carbon dioxide dissociation curves, drawn on the
same scales, showing relative linearity of the carbon dioxide
dissociation curve, compared with the sigmoid shape of the ODC,
which explains why carbon dioxide retention rarely arises from
$\dot{V}a/\dot{Q}$ imbalance

little effect on arterial $PO_2$, in contrast to the hypoxaemia resulting
from ventilation/perfusion imbalance. Again, however, as the arterial
venous difference in $PCO_2$ is usually only 0.4–1.0 kPa (3–7.5 mmHg), a
shunt ratio of less than 30% will have little effect on arterial $PCO_2$
values (see Chapter 3).

Although a restrictive pattern of respiratory function (low TLC and
VC, low RV/TLC ratio) is frequently associated with type I respiratory failure, the old idea that 'alveolar capillary block' caused the
hypoxaemia due to thickening of the alveolar–capillary membrane is
no longer tenable. In nearly all these cases hypoxaemia is due, in fact,
to increased variability of ventilation/perfusion ratios amongst different alveoli of the lungs.

*Diagnosis*

Diagnosis of type I respiratory failure clearly depends upon measurement of arterial blood gas tensions. A clinical clue to the possibility of

this is, of course, the recognition of central cyanosis, as shown by blueness of tongue, conjunctivae and warm mucous membranes.

The causes of type I respiratory failure involve most diseases which cause sufficient impairment of gas exchange in a large enough number of alveoli. These therefore include chronic bronchitis and emphysema, at an early stage before the development of hypoventilation complicates type I respiratory failure, so resulting in type II respiratory failure (see later); pneumonia; acute pulmonary oedema; pulmonary thromboembolism; an attack of bronchial asthma; collapse of a lobe or lobule; fibrosing and allergic alveolitis; and many other patterns of generalized lung disease. There is *no specific diagnostic implication* in the demonstration of type I respiratory failure, by finding hypoxaemia combined with a low or normal $P_{CO_2}$ on arterial blood gas estimation. The diagnosis can be achieved only by synthesis of the clinical, functional and radiographic features in each individual case. Nonetheless, the recognition of type I respiratory failure does carry implications for therapy.

## Treatment

Arterial hypoxaemia usually means that oxygen transport to the cells of the body, where oxygen is used in the mitochondria, is in peril. However, sufficient oxygen supply can still be guaranteed if the cardiac output is increased and/or the haemoglobin concentration or oxygen carrying capacity of the arterial blood is also increased. These physiological adaptations to hypoxaemia are usually adequate, but it will be clear that the combination of arterial hypoxaemia and a low fixed cardiac output is potentially very dangerous. This combination occurs, of course, in shock from any cause and is particularly lethal in cardiogenic shock, where pulmonary oedema, causing hypoxaemia, is combined with a low cardiac output. Failure of adequate oxygenation of the tissues is revealed by the presence of *lactic acidosis*, indicating failure of the biochemical mechanisms of energy supply, as there is insufficient oxygen to act as an adequate electron receptor in the redox linked reactions in the Kreb's tricarboxylic acid cycle in the cellular mitochondria (Fig. 54). As a consequence, metabolism of the primary food stuffs, carbohydrate, fat and protein, ceases at the level of acetyl coenzyme A with resultant formation of lactic acid. The resultant *metabolic acidosis* can be lethal. However, lactic acidosis is rarely found in chronic arterial hypoxaemia, as clearly the body cannot sustain for long a condition of inadequate cellular oxygenation.

High concentrations of inspired oxygen are used in treatment of type I respiratory failure; oxygen therapy is recommended when the arterial $P_{O_2}$ is persistently below 6.7 kPa (50 mmHg) and should aim to increase the arterial $P_{O_2}$ to at least 8.0 kPa (60 mmHg). If, however, the patient has a low cardiac output, as in myocardial infarction, haemorrhagic shock, severe pulmonary thromboembolism, etc., the

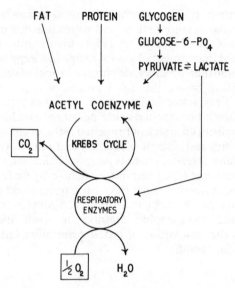

*Fig. 54.*    Biochemical use of oxygen, indicating that carbohydrate metabolism from glycogen is blocked at the stage of formation of
lactate if there is insufficient oxygen to allow the respiratory
enzymes linked to Kreb's cycle to function (*From D. C. Flenley
(1978) in Recent Advances in Respiratory Medicine I, ed. T. B.
Stretton. Edinburgh: Churchill Livingstone*)

inspired oxygen concentration should be raised to such a level to
achieve an arterial oxygen tension of at least 14 kPa (105 mmHg). This
can be achieved by high concentrations of oxygen, delivered by mask,
at a flow rate of 6 litres/minute (e.g. BOC Polymask, a tight-fitting
double plastic bag, fitted around the nose and lips which provides an
inspired oxygen concentration of around 60% at a flow rate of 6
litres/minute). An alternative is the MC mask, a similar tight-fitting
device which gives the same level of inspired oxygen concentration.
Some rebreathing of carbon dioxide occurs with these tight-fitting
masks, but this is irrelevant in this context, as the arterial $P_{CO_2}$ is
either low or at normal levels. However, patients tolerate any mask
badly and nasal prongs, projecting 1 cm or so into the anterior nares, at
a flow rate of 3 or even 4 litres of oxygen/minute can raise the inspired
oxygen concentration to around 40–50%, even although the patient
appears to breath through his mouth. Nonetheless, at these high flow
rates, there is some drying of the nasal mucosa. A useful compromise is
to give 2 litres of oxygen/minute by nasal prongs, at the same time as 6
litres of oxygen/minute by a tight-fitting mask, so that even if the

patient removes the mask for a short time he still has some enrichment of inspired oxygen. Furthermore, within such a mask the inspired oxygen concentration probably approaches 80% or more. These high concentrations are safe to administer to patients with *type I respiratory failure* as there is no risk of carbon dioxide retention from oxygen administration in such patients.

## Type II respiratory failure

In a normal subject a rise in arterial $PCO_2$ provokes an increase in ventilation, by central stimulation of the respiratory centres (see Chapter 4), so increasing breathing as to lower the $PCO_2$. In type II respiratory failure this mechanism has clearly failed, indicating that in addition to any lung disease, there is also abnormality of ventilatory control mechanisms. Clinical detection of type II respiratory failure is difficult. In practice the recognition of central cyanosis is a reliable guide to arterial hypoxaemia. If this sign is detected in a patient in whom type II respiratory failure is known to be a possibility, the diagnosis can only be accurately confirmed by measurement of arterial blood gas tensions. So-called *signs of carbon dioxide retention*, including tachycardia, distension of forearm veins, flapping irregular tremor of the outstretched hands, and clouding of consciousness, are all *unreliable* signs of carbon dioxide retention, as they can all have causes other than this condition. Furthermore, their absence does not preclude the presence of carbon dioxide retention.

### Causes

The causes of type II respiratory failure include chronic bronchitis and emphysema, particularly during an acute exacerbation (see Chapter 9); this is by far the commonest cause of carbon dioxide retention in adult medical practice. Type II respiratory failure can also arise in many other conditions, notably a severe attack of bronchial asthma, where a raised $PCO_2$ is an indication for consideration of mechanical ventilation; rarely in pulmonary oedema, notably that due to heroin overdosage; and in conditions affecting the chest wall or respiratory centres. Narcotic analgesics and other sedative drug overdoses can cause carbon dioxide retention associated with profound disturbance of consciousness. *Primary alveolar hypoventilation* is usually combined with obesity, such patients being specifically prone to develop *sleep apnoea* (see Chapter 24) of obstructive type. *Mechanical disorders* of the thoracic cage, such as scoliosis, fibro-thorax, anklyosing spondylitis or a late result of thoracoplasty, are all recognized causes of type II respiratory failure. *Neuromuscular diseases*, involving the muscles of the thoracic cage include polio-myelitis, amyotrophic lateral sclerosis, muscular dystrophy; spinal cord injury, multiple sclerosis, myasthenia gravis and peripheral neuropathy. Gas exchange in the lungs is also usually impaired. This results from the primary failure of the cough mechanism which characterizes the respiratory complications of these disorders, resulting in recurrent aspiration pneumonia.

*Treatment*

Treatment of type II respiratory failure depends upon recognition of its cause. In the common variety arising from an acute exacerbation of chronic bronchitis and emphysema, the basis of therapy is controlled oxygen therapy. This aims to provide sufficient oxygen to relieve the danger of death from hypoxaemia, without at the same time removing totally the respiratory drive resulting from hypoxaemia, which would then allow the arterial $P$CO$_2$ to rise, with the resultant fall in pH possibly killing the patient from respiratory acidosis. Recommendations for guidelines and management of this therapy are given in Chapter 9. Controlled oxygen therapy can be provided by nasal prongs, with oxygen at a flow rate of 1–2 litres/minute, adjusted according to the arterial $P$O$_2$ attained, or by the Edinburgh Mask at a flow rate of 2 litres/minute, or the 28% Ventimask, both of which provide roughly the same inspired oxygen concentration. However, in practice all masks are poorly tolerated and nasal prongs are the preferred method of providing controlled oxygen therapy to these patients.

Type II respiratory failure rising from *causes other than chronic bronchitis and emphysema* will usually be an indication for institution of mechanical ventilation. This is best provided by a cuffed endotracheal tube with intermittent positive pressure ventilation. The ventilator should be set so as to provide an adequate level of oxygenation (arterial $P$O$_2$ at least 8.0 kPa; 60 mmHg), without excessive fall in arterial $P$CO$_2$, which should best be maintained above 4.0 kPa (30 mmHg). Prolonged mechanical ventilation with an inspired oxygen concentration above 40% carries the risk of inducing *lung damage from oxygen*, one of the causes of the adult respiratory distress syndrome (see Chapter 21).

# The adult respiratory distress syndrome

In 1967 the term adult respiratory distress syndrome was coined to describe patients in whom breathlessness, severe hypoxaemia and bilateral infiltrates in the chest radiograph developed some 24–72 hours after non-thoracic trauma or pancreatitis. At autopsy (for nearly all died), the lungs were like liver, with a protein-rich oedema fluid filling alveoli, leaving a few air-filled spaces lined by a hyaline membrane, reminiscent of that seen in the respiratory distress syndrome of the neonate. Despite earlier controversy, the term is now widely used throughout the world, it being agreed that this clinical and pathophysiological entity has many different causes.

## Causes

The causes of ARDS include:

1. Pneumonia, due to bacterial (*Strep. pneumoniae*, staphylococci, *Klebsiella*, etc.) viral or fungal pathogens (see Chapter 8).

2. Trauma, often not primarily involving the thorax, as for example in fat embolism or hypotensive shock ('shock lung').

3. Disseminated infection causing sepsis, particularly from Gram-negative bacteraemia.

4. Chemical pneumonitis, as from aspiration of gastric acid (pH < 3.0), near drowning (see Chapter 8) and inhalation of smoke or chemical irritants (nitrous oxide, phosgene, etc.), and pulmonary oxygen toxicity from prolonged administration of high concentrations of inspired oxygen.

5. Drug overdosage and poisoning; as with heroin, salicylates, barbiturates or the weed-killer paraquat (see Chapter 21).

6. Miscellaneous causes include acute pancreatitis, disseminated intravascular coagulation, air or amniotic fluid embolism and cerebral trauma (neurogenic pulmonary oedema) (see Chapter 22).

Pneumonia is the commonest cause in civilian practice, but the term 'shock lung' (ARDS due to non-thoracic trauma), leaped to prominence during the Vietnam War, possibly as helicopter transport and intense resuscitation allowed casualties to live long enough to develop this desperate complication.

## Pathogenesis

The fundamental pathological abnormality in adult respiratory distress syndrome seems to be disruption of the alveolar capillary membrane, with resultant exudation of a protein-rich oedema fluid into alveoli and interstitial spaces. Fibrinogen then degrades alveolar surfactant causing atelectasis, so that eventually the only air-containing spaces are alveolar ducts lined with hyaline membrane (Fig. 55) composed of intra-alveolar organization of fibrinogen. Alveolar epithelium bears the brunt of the damage; surprisingly, the capillary endothelium may seem to be intact, despite evidence that it has allowed leak of high molecular weight protein molecules from the plasma. Hyperplasia of alveolar type II cells yield the new epithelial lining, eventually transforming into the flat type I cells forming the alveolar epithelium of the regenerated air spaces. Microemboli of platelets and fibrin are prominent in the capillaries.

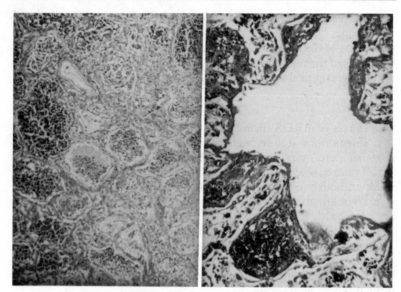

*Fig. 55.*    Autopsy appearances of lung from a case of the adult respiratory
distress syndrome, showing the complete filling of some alveoli,
and in others the formation of a hyaline membrane, with
disorganized air spaces and greatly thickened alveolar walls

Mechanisms damaging the alveolar capillary membrane must
clearly vary, dependent upon the cause of adult respiratory distress
syndrome. Emboli composed of aggregated polymorphs, following
complement activation, may damage the epithelium when these
phagocytes release their activated oxygen, which is normally reserved
for killing phagocytosed bacteria (see Chapter 2). Platelet emboli may
release kinins and histamine, but despite much experimental work the
exact pathogenesis remains obscure. Rational prevention of the adult
respiratory distress syndrome must therefore await elucidation of
these as yet unknown mechanisms.

## Clinical features

Adult respiratory distress syndrome classically arises after a latent
period of 24–72 hours following a catastrophic acute disease. The
lungs, which have previously been normal before the insult, give
evidence of their involvement by the slow development of breathlessness, with rapid shallow breathing and central cyanosis. Anxiety and
restlessness are common, but may well be attributed to the primary
disease such as non-thoracic multiple trauma, etc.

Arterial blood gas analysis will confirm the presence of hypoxaemia
with a widened alveolar to arterial oxygen tension gradient ($A\text{-}aDO_2$) to

a value greater than 3.3 kPa (25 mmHg). The $P_{CO_2}$ is often low, at least initially, the patient therefore suffering from type I respiratory failure. Furthermore, this hypoxaemia is relatively refractory to oxygen therapy, for example with an inspired oxygen concentration of 60% (Polymask or MC mask at 6 litres of oxygen/minute), the arterial $P_{O_2}$ will often remain below 6.7 kPa (50 mmHg) in the established syndrome. This indicates that the shunt fraction is increased, commonly to values as high as 50% or more. To quantitate the shunt more precisely, 95% oxygen (balance nitrogen) is given (see Fig. 16), but by this time the patient will usually be receiving mechanical ventilation. 100% oxygen is avoided in this circumstance, as this gas is potentially 100% absorbable, so carrying a grave risk of increasing the collapse of alveoli which already have a very low ventilation–perfusion ratio. The *chest radiograph* usually shows diffuse bilateral infiltrations, which characteristically spare the periphery of the lungs and the costophrenic angles. These opacities are readily apparent at the stage when the arterial $P_{O_2}$ is reduced in ARDS.

## Special investigations

A flow-directed balloon-tipped Swan-Ganz catheter can measure both pulmonary arterial and wedge pressures and also allow measurement of the cardiac output by thermal dilution technique, these measurements being made in the intensive care unit. In patients with established adult respiratory distress syndrome the cardiac output is either normal or raised and the pulmonary arterial pressure is also high, but the pulmonary capillary pressure is normal. The cardiac output falls as the syndrome progresses, and carbon dioxide retention may be a terminal event, coupled with systemic hypotension and very low cardiac output, with severe and refractory arterial hypoxaemia. During mechanical ventilation the lungs characteristically appear to be very stiff (low compliance), so that high inspiratory pressures are necessary to generate an adequate tidal volume.

## Differential diagnosis

A latent period, without respiratory symptoms following the initial event, occurring before the development of acute respiratory disturbance, is characteristic of ARDS. If this history is not obtained, adult respiratory distress syndrome must be distinguished from:

1. Pulmonary oedema, where the usual cardiogenic origin is often myocardial infarction, or over-hydration (see Chapter 22).

2. Bilateral aspiration pneumonia, particularly if the cough mechanism has failed (see Chapter 2).

3. Multiple pulmonary infarction, where a source of pulmonary emboli may be found (see Chapter 18).

Adult respiratory distress syndrome is clearly not an aetiological diagnosis and use of the term should not inhibit the search for a cause, which may require specific treatment (e.g. bacterial pneumonia), in addition to the supportive treatment which is all that can be offered for the syndrome itself.

## Treatment

The development of adult respiratory distress syndrome may be prevented if the primary condition is adequately treated, e.g. shock corrected, aspiration avoided and over-enthusiastic intravenous infusion of crystalloids discouraged. Whole blood is the best replacement for blood loss and it must be recognized that infusion of large volumes of crystalloids is potentially dangerous in patients in whom plasma protein levels are initially low or in those at risk of having developed damage to the alveolar capillary membrane. Mechanical ventilation may have been instituted as part of the treatment of the primary cause of the syndrome. This may be accelerated by ventilator-induced lung damage, which can be avoided if a volume-cycled machine is used, set to have a tidal volume of around 10–12 ml/kg/body weight, the respiratory rate being adjusted to keep the arterial $P_{CO_2}$ in the normal range, and *not* with excessive ventilation and a low $P_{CO_2}$.

*Lung damage from oxygen*, first described experimentally in a cat 180 years ago, poses a problem in the management and prevention of adult respiratory distress syndrome. Such patients are hypoxic and the hypoxia is characteristically refractory to an increase in the inspired oxygen concentration. If a normal subject breathes an inspired oxygen concentration of 50% or higher for more than 24–48 hours, substernal tightness and cough are then combined with a fall in vital capacity, and if the inhalation continues without interruption by periods of breathing air, the high level of inspired oxygen can itself lead to adult respiratory distress syndrome. This therapeutic dilemma, whereby life-giving oxygen may further damage the lungs, so as to require yet a further increase in inspired oxygen to maintain an adequate arterial $P_{O_2}$, has not been fully resolved. If the cardiac output is normal, and the metabolic demands of the patient for oxygen not grossly raised by fever, hypoxic death can probably be prevented if the $P_{O_2}$ is kept at around 6.7 kPa (50 mmHg), if the haemoglobin concentration is normal. Inspired oxygen concentrations higher than that necessary to achieve this $P_{O_2}$ should thus be avoided for continual treatment of any patient with potential or established ARDS. If this cannot be achieved without an inspired oxygen concentration of over 50% in a patient receiving mechanical ventilation, a positive end-expiratory pressure (PEEP) of at first 5 cmH$_2$O should be tried, to see if this can achieve the desired arterial $P_{O_2}$. PEEP unfortunately impedes venous return and so lowers the cardiac output, and a trial-and-error manipulation of

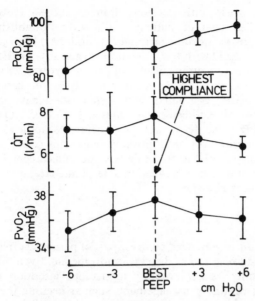

*Fig. 56.*    Relationship of respiratory compliance (pressure required to produce a given volume of inflation at the end of an inspiratory cycle), cardiac output QT and mixed venous oxygen tension ($PvO_2$), measured from an indwelling pulmonary arterial catheter, in a patient with ARDS at different levels of PEEP. Increase of PEEP reduces cardiac output, and although raising arterial $PO_2$ may reduce mixed venous oxygen tension (so that an optimal setting is required) (*From Suter et al.(1976) New England Journal of Medicine, 292, 286*)

the level of PEEP against the mixed venous $PO_2$ (obtained from a Swan-Ganz pulmonary arterial catheter) may be used in a sophisticated intensive care unit, where such patients should be treated (Fig. 56).

Corticosteroids may have a role in preventing the development of the syndrome when used in massive doses, simply by inhibiting the activation of complement, with the resultant damage to the alveolar capillary membrane, but these drugs are useless once the syndrome has become established. Similarly, diuretics (in the absence of cardiogenic pulmonary oedema) are useless, as is heparinization of the patient.

*Extracorporeal membrane oxygenation* (ECMO) aims to sustain life by providing oxygen and removing carbon dioxide from the blood stream by an artificial external membrane lung, fed by an extracorporeal circulation. This treatment, possibly the most expensive of all in high-technology medicine, has been used in over 200 patients throughout the world, with occasional dramatic success. However, in a recent controlled trial of patients with severe established adult respiratory distress syndrome (arterial $PO_2$ under 6.7 kPa (50 mmHg) when being ventilated with 100% inspired oxygen at 5 cm PEEP) failed to show any improvement in survival of patients treated with ECMO, when compared to those treated conventionally by mechanical ventilation with PEEP, combined with other supportive measures. However, recently it has been suggested that partial ECMO may be of value in treating these desperately ill patients. Nonetheless, as with heart transplantation, research into improving this costly method of treatment seems justifiable only in a few specialized centres and the treatment cannot be recommended in a desperate attempt to save life by the casual user elsewhere.

## Prognosis

Even in the most experienced centres, 50% of patients suffering from established adult respiratory distress syndrome die. Even this level of survival can only be achieved by meticulous attention to detail, particularly in ventilator management, such as keeping the inspired oxygen concentration below 50%, scrupulous asepsis in management of ventilators, humidifiers and suctioning equipment, and avoiding the continuous use of high levels of PEEP. Full restoration of normal respiratory function may be regained only very slowly after severe adult respiratory distress syndrome.

## Further reading

BERGOFSKY, E. H. (1979) Respiratory failure in disorders of the thoracic cage. *Am. Rev. resp. Dis.*, **119**, 643–669.
FLENLEY, D. C. and WARREN, P. M. (1980) Chronic bronchitis and emphysema. In *Recent Advances in Respiratory Medicine II*, ed. D. C. Flenley. Edinburgh: Churchill Livingstone.
MODELL, J. H. (1978) Biology of drowning. *A. Rev. Med.*, **29**, 1–8.
MURRAY, J. F. (1980) Adult respiratory distress syndrome. In *Recent Advances in Respiratory Medicine II*, ed. D. C. Flenley. Edinburgh: Churchill Livingstone.
SYKES, M. K., McNICOL, M. W. and CAMPBELL, E. J. M. (1976) *Respiratory Failure*, 2nd ed. Oxford: Blackwell Scientific.

# 12

# Bronchiectasis, Lung Abscess and Cystic Fibrosis

## Bronchiectasis

Bronchiectasis is defined as persistent dilatation of bronchi. This can only be proved to be present in life by bronchography, where the bronchial mucosa is outlined by a radio-opaque material. The incidence of bronchiectasis in developed countries has fallen following the widespread use of antibiotics to treat respiratory infections, but it remains a common problem in the developing countries.

### Causes

Causes of bronchiectasis, from congenital to acquired, include:

1. A congenital anatomical abnormality, notably an *intrapulmonary lung sequestration*, where a detached portion of non-functioning lung exists, which receives a blood supply directly from the aorta, but with venous drainage into the pulmonary veins. If the sequestered segment communicates with the bronchial tree, infection eventually results, the cystic spaces becoming filled with pus. Clinically presenting with a pneumonia, often in an adult, the true nature of the sequestration is revealed as the chest radiograph clears to show a localized mass of cysts, with or without fluid levels, most often lying in the posterior basal region of the left lower lobe. The cysts do not fill on bronchography.

2. *Hypogammaglobulinaemia*, which can be due to the rare congenital form, transmitted as an X-linked genetic disease, the affected boys having no B lymphocytes and therefore tiny tonsils. The commoner type of *varied agammaglobulinaemia* (acquired or of late onset) affects both sexes. In these patients the B cells fail to transform into immunoglobulin-secreting plasma cells, so that the serum IgG is less than 250 mg/dl, and IgA and IgM are less than 50 mg/dl. Autoimmune pernicious anaemia is a recognized association, as is nodular lymphoid hyperplasia of the gut, with chronic diarrhoea, sprue and intestinal giardiasis.

3. *Kartagener's syndrome* (situs inversus, chronic sinusitis and bronchiectasis), which occurs in about 1 in 30 000 Caucasians. About

half of these will also have the *immotile cilia syndrome*, which is always associated with male sterility. Respiratory tract (and other) cilia have the same ultrastructural basis of their motility as that seen on electron microscopy in the tails of spermatozoa. In this syndrome the dynein arms which allow this movement can be shown to be missing on electron microscopy. Clinically recurrent pneumonia and bronchiectasis are common from childhood, being associated with recurrent maxillary sinusitis and failure of development of the frontal sinuses. Otitis media and deafness are common. Chronic bronchitis complicates the bronchiectasis and respiratory mucociliary clearancy is severely impaired. Not all patients with the immotile cilia syndrome have situs inversus, in which the major organs have a mirror image reversal in the body, with dextrocardia etc. The prognosis of both syndromes is reasonably good if smoking is avoided and the recurrent respiratory infections are promptly treated.

4. A *late sequela of chronic infection*, notably in post-primary pulmonary tuberculosis, where bronchiectasis is commonly found if bronchograms are carried out, particular with upper lobe lesions. However, the disease is symptomatic only if lower lobes are involved, in some cases following primary pulmonary tuberculosis, with persistent segmental shadows at the time of primary infection. Pneumonia in infancy, due to measles or whooping cough, or possibly bronchiolitis due to respiratory syncitial virus infection, may all be followed by subsequent bronchiectasis in later life.

5. *Bronchial obstruction* by a foreign body or adenoma can lead to bronchiectasis as a result of infection 'behind the block'.

6. *Allergic bronchopulmonary aspergillosis*, with asthma, eosinophilia of both blood and sputum, and fleeting segmental opacities on the chest radiograph due to transient collapse behind mucous plugs which contain aspergillus mycelia. *Aspergillus fumigatus* may be seen in the sputum and the mucous plugs and may also be grown on sputum culture. Precipitins to *Aspergillus* are invariably present in the serum, and immediate skin tests to *A. fumigatus* extracts are positive. Upper or lower lung lobes may be involved in the bronchiectasis, which characteristically involves the *proximal portions* of the bronchi, with relatively normal distal bronchi, whereas in all other patterns of bronchiectasis the major site of dilatation is in the distal bronchi.

## Pathology

The bronchial dilatation may be *saccular*, with cysts which can extend to the pleural surface. They are lined by squamous or columnar epithelium, with little evidence of normal bronchial anatomy. Less severe destruction occurs in *cylindrical* or *varicose* bronchiectasis, but again the bronchial wall is infiltrated by neutrophils and the adjoining lung may show collapse, pneumonia and/or fibrosis. The bronchial arteries in the bronchiectatic segments are hypertrophied and increased in number, with prominent pre-capillary communication, transferring blood from the bronchial to the pulmonary circulation, so that pulmonary hypertension is a recognized complication of extensive bronchiectasis.

## Pathogenesis

Repeated bronchial infection is both the cause and effect of the bronchial dilatation. The primary abnormality is clearly a breach in the respiratory defences against infection (see Chapter 2), either by immunoglobulin deficiency, impaired mucociliary clearance or local mechanical obstruction or following a virulent pneumonia in childhood. The weakened bronchial walls then dilate in response to the constant negative intrapleural pressure, and so further impair the efficiency of mucociliary clearance. Bacterial pathogens found in the sputum include anaerobes (including Vincent's organisms, particularly in the untreated patient), but infection with *H. influenzae* and *Strep. pneumoniae*, streptococci and staphylococci is more usual in patients who have received antibiotics from time to time.

## Clinical features

Cough, with large volumes of persistently purulent sputum, and intermittent *haemoptysis* are the characteristic features. Profuse haemoptysis without purulent sputum (*bronchiectasis haemorrhagica sicca*) is well recognized and is presumed to arise from the distended veins or from the dilated bronchopulmonary anastomoses. Breathlessness is related to the accompanying chronic bronchitis, which is shown by a persistently low $FEV_1$.

Finger-clubbing occurs in over 30% of cases and areas of localized crepitations over the affected segments are usual during an exacerbation. Rhonchi, with or without audible wheeze, are of course characteristic of asthma due to allergic bronchopulmonary aspergillosis. *Brain abscess* and *amyloidosis* are rare but recognized complications of bronchiectasis of any origin.

The *chest radiograph* can be normal, but more often shows streaky infiltrates, particularly in the lower zones if the cavities are filled with pus. In advanced saccular disease ring-shaped shadows, with or without fluid levels, may be seen. Bronchial wall thickening in allergic bronchopulmonary aspergillosis can show as 'tram-lines', radiating from the hilum, or as circular ring shadows. The diagnosis of bronchiectasis is proved by *bronchography* (Fig. 57), which should only be carried out after postural drainage and antibiotic therapy have cleared secretions. Bronchography can precipitate a severe attack in an asthmatic patient and, if it is indicated in such a patient, should

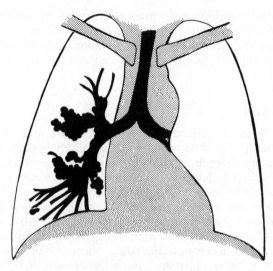

*Fig. 57.*    Bronchogram of the right lung, in a patient with cystic bronchiectasis, showing filling of the cystic bronchiectatic cavities in the
middle lobe and the basal segments of the lower lobe

therefore always be preceded by adequate steroid therapy and other
bronchodilators. Bronchoscopy can often be usefully combined with
bronchography, so as to determine the site of any haemoptysis and also
to search for a foreign body. Selective bronchography, however, is
rarely practicable through the narrow channels of the fibreoptic
bronchoscope, which become clogged by the viscid bronchographic
media. The radio-opaque material can be injected through a catheter
passed through the nose, under local anaesthesia, the catheter then
being screened so as to lie in the appropriate main bronchus. Breathing
and coughing are encouraged as 2–3 ml of medium are injected every
four or five expiratory movements, to a total dose of 12–15 ml.
Alternatively, bronchography can be carried out under general
anaesthesia, when combined with bronchoscopy, particularly if the
rigid bronchoscope is employed. The bronchi in both lungs (possibly
visualized at two separate sessions) must be seen if surgical treatment
is contemplated.

*Respiratory function* may be normal in localized bronchiectasis, but
many patients show an obstructive pattern, which is partly reversible
with steroids in allergic bronchopulomary aspergillosis, but relatively
irreversible in the more common accompanying chronic bronchitis
and emphysema. Hypoxaemia is usual if airways obstruction is
prominent.

*The defence mechanisms* of the respiratory tract are assessed by
measurements of serum immunoglobulins, *Aspergillus* precipitins,

and the sweat sodium test for cystic fibrosis (see later). An increase in serum IgG, IgA or IgM has commonly been found in those patients with bronchiectasis who do not have hypogammaglobulinaemia, this presumably representing a chronic response to the persistence of bacterial antigen.

## Treatment

*Postural drainage* uses gravity with assisted coughing and chest wall percussion to drain secretions from the affected lobe. This lobe must therefore be placed uppermost. This usually involves raising the foot of the bed if the lower lobes are affected, for at least 15 minutes twice daily, or for longer if the secretions are profuse. A trained physiotherapist then percusses over the affected lobe and ensures that that lobe is uppermost, and should also teach the patient's relatives how to carry out these manoeuvres.

*Antibiotics* are used to control infection. Ampicillin, 250 mg four times a day, will control the common *H. influenzae* and *Strep. pneumoniae* infections, but tetracycline 500 mg four times a day is also of proved value. It may be used to alternate with ampicillin in 10–14-day courses of each throughout a winter, possibly adding co-trimaxozole in a 14-day period, thus providing a cyclical regimen of anti-infective agents with the three drugs used sequentially.

*Surgical resection* of an affected lobe or segment is used relatively rarely today, although it can cure localized disease. Severe symptoms, strictly localized disease and otherwise good respiratory function are all indications for surgical resection, but they rarely coexist. Failure of postural drainage and antibiotics to control the disease adequately is often associated with poor respiratory function or generalized disease, both of which preclude surgery. Massive haemoptysis which cannot be controlled by local measures at bronchoscopy may demand emergency surgery to safe life.

*Agammaglobulinaemia* is treated by 100 mg/kg of immune serum globulin given every four weeks by intramuscular injection. Intravenous preparations, which may be more effective, as well as less painful and with better opsonising ability, are being evaluated.

*Allergic bronchopulmonary aspergillosis* requires the usual bronchodilators for the asthma, coupled with steroids by mouth (see Chapter 10). Unfortunately, doses up to 30 mg prednisolone/day may be needed to control the asthma and to inhibit progression of the bronchiectatic damage. This dose should be reduced to an acceptable 10 mg/day as soon as the exacerbation is over. Bronchoscopic aspiration of a mycelial plug causing atelectasis may be needed if it is not coughed out spontaneously.

The *prognosis* is good if the treatment outlined above is used. Surgery can offer cure, but the indications for successful resection are limited. Medical treatment is presumed to be life-long, but in most cases this can probably ensure that this patient's life is indeed long.

# Lung abscess

Lung abscess means local destruction of lung tissue by pyogenic organisms. Lung abscess can be caused by:

1. *Aspiration pneumonia*, which can progress to abscess formation (see Chapter 8), this being a well recognized complication of inhalation of a foreign body. Lung abscess is a traditional hazard of dental extraction if an infected tooth lodges in a bronchus. Anaerobic infection is particularly common in inhalational lung abscess, often causing the sputum to have a foul smell.

2. *Blockage of a bronchus* by tumour or foreign body, which can be followed by an intense suppurative pneumonia behind the block, with abscess formation.

3. *Pneumonia*, particularly *Staphylococcus pyogenes* (see Chapter 8), *Klebsiella*, and legionnaire's disease, all of which are recognized causes of lung abscess.

4. *Infected pulomonary infarction*, rarely from a septic thrombus, or from presumed bacterial inhalation into an already infarcted area.

5. *Trauma* to the lung. In amoebiasis a right-sided pleural effusion may be associated with an amoebic abscess in the right lower lobe, as a result of transdiaphragmatic spread from hepatic amoebiasis.

## Clinical features

Aspiration pneumonia, particularly in the hospitalized patient, can progress to lung abscess with little systemic disturbance. However, fever and rigors are more classical features and are usually associated with cough and localized pleuritic chest pain. The diagnostic expectoration of a large volume of foul-smelling blood-stained pus, as the abscess bursts into a bronchus, is today usually prevented by antibiotic therapy, which may turn an acute process into a chronic thick-walled cavity. Pleural effusion and empyema may well be associated. Rupture of the abscess cavity into the pleural space is associated with severe pleuritic pain, which results in the formation of a pyopneumothorax, with a fluid level indicating the presence of both gas and fluid in the pleural space.

Diminished movement, dullness to percussion and impaired breath sounds over the affected lesion are usual, with signs of a cavity being rare. Clubbing of the fingers can develop rapidly and fluctuation of the nail beds may be prominent.

The white blood count classically shows a polymorphonuclear leucocytosis. The sputum contains many pus cells, usually with a mixed bacterial flora. In aspiration pneumonia anaerobic bacteria may be present, but are revealed only by appropriate culture methods.

The *chest radiograph* initially shows pneumonic consolidation, later progressing to the characteristic cavity, often with a fluid level, which provides the diagnosis. However, lung abscess must be distinguished from *other cavitated lesions* in the chest radiograph. Other less common causes of this appearance include:

1. *Congenital*: bronchogenic cysts usually in the medial third of the lower lobes.

2. *Infective*: actinomycosis, with great destruction in the lower lobes being associated with empyema and possibly periostial reaction in overlying ribs; hydatid cysts in the lower lobes, sometimes with the 'water-lily' sign; rare fungal infections such as coccidioidomycosis.

3. *Immunological*: Wegener's granulomatosis; necrobiotic rheumatoid nodules, which are usually multiple (see Chapter 19).

4. *Neoplastic* cavitated secondary deposits and Hodgkin's disease.

5. *Occupational*: complicated coal-worker's pneumoconiosis and silicosis (see Chapter 17).

The two commonest causes of a cavitated pulmonary lesions, other than lung abscess, are *tuberculosis*, particularly involving the upper lobes, but only very rarely showing a fluid level, and usually with some bilateral disease; and a *cavitated squamous bronchial carcinoma* (see Chapter 14). As with other chronic pyogenic pulmonary infection, cerebral abscess and amyloidosis are both recognized complications of lung abscess.

## Treatment

Antibiotics are essential. The organism may not be known initially, particularly in a lung abscess resulting from aspiration. Intramuscular benzylpenicillin in a dose of at least 2 megaunits daily may be combined with ampicillin (500 mg four times daily by mouth), combined with metronidazole (400 mg three times daily by mouth), which will cover the probable infections with a mixed flora of aerobic and anaerobic bacteria. Antibiotic therapy for staphylococcal, pneumococcal and *Legionella* pneumonia is discussed in Chapter 8.

Postural drainage, with percussion over the affected area by a physiotherapist, may help to drain the abscess. Drainage by bronchoscopy has traditionally relied upon the rigid bronchoscope, but recently success has been achieved by an ingenious adaptation of the fibreoptic bronchoscope, whereby a Swan-Ganz catheter is passed through the fibrescope into the affected segmental bronchus. The balloon of the catheter is then inflated, so opening the abscess cavity, but preventing aspiration of the abscess contents throughout the bronchial tree, which was formerly a recognized serious hazard of any attempt to drain the abscess intrabronchially.

Surgical resection by lobectomy may be required if a chronic abscess cannot be otherwise drained, or to remove destroyed lung which is impairing respiratory function. Empyema complicating a lung abscess or a pyopneumothorax may require surgical drainage.

# Cystic fibrosis

Cystic fibrosis is the commonest Mendelian genetic disorder in Caucasians, occurring in about one in 2000 births in Europe and North America, but the disease is very rare in Asians and Africans. It is inherited as an autosomal recessive, so that both the patient's parents must carry the gene, and there is a one in four chance that other children of these parents will be affected. The cystic fibrosis gene may in future be detected by the presence of a newly described serum lectin, present in both patients (homozygotes) and probably in carriers (heterozygotes).

Paediatricians encounter cystic fibrosis as a cause of meconium ileus in the neonate, and later pancreatic insufficiency with failure to thrive, and still later as recurrent respiratory tract infections and persistent productive cough with wheeze and clubbing. However, with modern continued care, physiotherapy and antibiotics, many of these patients now survive to adolescence and beyond, and it is the problems of these adult patients which are discussed particularly in this chapter.

## Pathology

The fundamental defect remains unknown, but may rest in the glycoprotein components of the cell membrane, which affect the ability to transport calcium intracellularly. Exocrine gland secretions have a reduced water content, and this includes the bronchial mucous glands, so that the very viscid secretions that are produced tend to plug small airways. The submucosal bronchial glands are hypertrophied, and these primarily viscid secretions are always infected, so that the secretions are purulent, and the airways inflamed. The infection is mainly a bronchiolitis, with areas of bronchial stenosis and obliteration, which produces airway obstruction and inhibits the growth of the lungs. Panacinar emphysema also contributes to the disorganization of lung structure, which eventually leads to hypoxia. Pulmonary arterial walls are then thickened and eventually right ventricular hypertrophy develops.

The *pancreas* is usually fibrosed, diabetes developing in up to 10% of adult patients. Recurrent attacks of acute pancreatitis can occur. Faecal impaction can cause intestinal obstruction and gall stones with abnormalities of the gall bladder are common. Cirrhosis of the liver, sometimes with portal hypertension, can affect some 5% of those patients surviving to adult life.

## Clinical features

Cough, with purulent copious sputum and frequent haemoptysis (in up to 50% of adults), is a dominant symptom. As in bronchiectasis, breathlessness is more related to concomitant airways obstruction, as shown by a low $FEV_1$, and is rarely a major feature. Finger-clubbing is almost invariable, but hypertrophic pulmonary osteoarthropathy is uncommon. The chest shows hyperflation with variable crepitations and wheezing. Spontaneous pneumothorax is a recognized complication.

The *chest radiograph* confirms the hyperinflation, with a long thin heart, and parallel shadows (or 'tram-lines') with thickened bronchi and nodular and ring shadows, but occasionally with large dense opacities.

The *sputum* contains *Staph. pyogenes*, *H. influenzae* and *Pseudomonas aeruginosa* as the main pathogens, mucoid strains of *Pseudomonas* being particularly common in the adult.

The *sweat test* is diagnostic, if the pilocarpine ionotophoresis method is used on a sample of at least 50 mg of sweat. Although sodium and chloride concentrations over 60 mmol/litre are diagnostic of cystic fibrosis in children, values above 65–70 mmol/litres are probably needed to confirm the diagnosis in the adult. Furthermore, in equivocal cases, it is noteworthy that these concentrations do not fall in response to oral fludrocortisone.

*Respiratory function tests* at first show an increase in closing volume, with expiratory flow rates being reduced at the lower lung volumes, as shown by the flow–volume curve. These results both suggest involvement of small airways. Later an obstructive pattern develops, with hyperinflation (high TLC, high RV/TLC ratio, low VC), and low $FEV_1$ and $FEV_1$/FVC ratio. Hypoxaemia is also more common in advanced cases, but a high $PCO_2$ is uncommon until the last stage associated with cor pulmonale.

### Extrapulmonary manifestations

Puberty is usually delayed, but most patients eventually grow to a normal height. Men are infertile and amenorrhoea often ensues in female patients. Pancreatic insufficiency is less prominent in those who survive to adult life and can be controlled by oral pancreatic enzymes (pancreatin), dietary fat restriction and vitamin supplements. *Meconium ileus*, with diarrhoea preceding an attack of colicky pain of intestinal obstruction, is a well recognized complication in the adult patient with cystic fibrosis. A mass can then be felt in the right iliac fossa, and the abdominal radiograph shows multiple fluid levels in the small bowel. Surgical treatment should be avoided and the condition usually responds to intravenous fluids, nasal suction and pancreatin.

*Diabetes* occurs in up to 10% of adult patients with cystic fibrosis.

Psychosocial disturbances are important, for these patients are often intelligent, but the need for continuous treatment often breeds an immature personality and jobs may be very difficult to find when a potential employer learns of the diagnosis.

## Treatment

As in bronchiectasis, the pulmonary condition responds best to a combination of postural drainage to clear secretions and antibiotics to control infection. The bases of the lungs are most often involved and thus the patient should be taught to cough with the head down, assisted by percussion over the basis by a trained relative, for up to four times a day so as to clear purulent secretions. These sessions of postural coughing should last for up to 15 minutes. Patients can also be taught to use the new technique of one or two forced expirations — a 'huff', during expiration from mid-lung volume down to low lung volume; the 'huffs' are combined with sharp adduction of the upper arm. This manoeuvre can be carried out by the patients themselves without assistance, and when it is followed by a few minutes of relaxed diaphragmatic breathing, and then by coughing, it has been shown to raise as much sputum as physiotherapist-assisted postural drainage. The ability to clear the chest for themselves using this 'huffing' technique greatly increases the patients' independence.

Some patients find that a five or 10-minute period of inhaling a saline aerosol, with or without a bronchodilator (e.g. terbutaline respiratory solution, 10 mg/ml) from a compressor-driven nebulizer, can liquefy secretions and thus make raising of sputum more effective.

*Antibiotics* should be used continuously, with selection guided by the current bacterial population of the sputum. Staphylococcal infection can usually be controlled by flucloxacillin or clindamycin, given in a high dosage early in an infective episode, when it has most ability to penetrate into the sputum. Amoxycillin, ampicillin and co-trimoxazole can all be used for *H. influenzae*, but many believe that chloramphenicol, which is active against both *Staph. pyogenes* and *H. influenzae*, is often the most effective oral antibiotic.

*Pseudomonas aeruginosa* is often resistant to many of the above agents, but seven to ten days of treatment with intramuscular gentamicin, so as to give a peak serum level of 5–100 $\mu$g/ml, with intravenous carbenicillin (20 g/day), is only justified if there is evidence that the infection is causing clinical deterioration or further functional impairment. Lower doses of these two drugs may be effective if inhaled as an aerosol twice daily. It is possible that the new antibiotic tobramycin may be preferable to gentamicin in treatment of *Pseudomonas* infections. Controlled trials to establish a firm basis for antibiotic usage are badly needed in cystic fibrosis, but are very difficult to carry out in such patients.

*Airways obstruction* sometimes responds to bronchodilators, including corticosteroids, and in some of these patients *Aspergillus fumigatus* has been isolated, and aspergillin precipitins found in the serum. Persistent hypoxaemia is usually a late development and the role of long-term oxygen therapy in these patients has not been assessed.

There is little doubt that the best results in treating these patients over the whole of their lives have been obtained when treatment is supervised from a special centre where medical, bacteriological and nursing care can be combined with expert physiotherapy and social work.

## Prognosis

It is only in the last 20 years that significant numbers of patients with cystic fibrosis have survived to adolescence, so that clearly experience with the disease in the adult phase is too recent for prognostic certainty. Nonetheless, it appears that the outlook is worse for those with persistent *Pseudomonas* infection, severe clinical disease and large volumes of sputum. Poor respiratory function, low body weight and older age at presentation do not appear to be related to the chance of early death. In a recent British study, the complications of diabetes, meconium ileus and spontaneous pneumothorax did not occur more often in those patients who died early, when compared to those who survived for prolonged periods.

## Further reading

AFZELIUS, B. A. and MOSSBERG, B. (1980) Immotile cilia. *Thorax*, **35**, 401–404.
LANDING, B. H. and DIXON, L. G. (1979) Congenital malformations and genetic disorders of the respiratory tract (larynx, trachea, bronchi and lungs). *Am. Rev. resp. Dis.*, **120**, 151–185.
MITCHELL-HEGGS, P., MEARNS, M. and BATTEN, J. C. (1976) Cystic fibrosis in adolescents and adults. *Q. Jl Med.*, **45**, 479–504.
DI SANT' AGNESE, P. A. and DAVIS, P. B. (1979) Cystic fibrosis in adults. 75 cases and review of 232 cases in the literature. *Am. J. Med.*, **66**, 121–132.
WOOD, R. E., BOAT, T. F. and DOERSHUK, C. F. (1976) Cystic fibrosis; state of the art. *Am. Rev. resp. Dis.*, **113**, 833–878.
YOSHIKAWA, T. T., CHOW, A. W. and GUZE, L. B. (1980) *Infectious Diseases: Diagnosis and Management.* Boston: Houghton Mifflin.

# 13

# Tuberculosis

As the words phthisis (to waste away) and haemoptysis (to spit blood) imply, tuberculosis was known to the Greeks before Hippocrates, but recognition that it was the disease resulting from infection with *Mycobacterium tuberculosis* had to await the microscope, aniline dyes and the genius of Robert Koch in 1882.

## Epidemiology

Tuberculosis was a great killer in antiquity, but really became 'captain of the men of death' when the industrial revolution herded folk into the great cities, to live huddled in the 'nests of tuberculosis', so graphically described by Sir Robert Philip. Improvement in these social conditions, combined with separation of the infectious patients, started the impressive decline of tuberculosis deaths seen from 1880 to 1940, when specific antituberculous drugs were first used (Fig. 58). Today the annual risk of tuberculosis infection in developed countries lies between 100 and 300 per 100 000, a rate which is halving every five to seven years (Figs 59, 60). Whereas in 1940 around 60% of the population of such developed countries had been infected at some time with *M. tuberculosis*, this fell to 25% of the population by 1975, and by the year 2000 it seems likely that only 5% of these populations will ever have been infected by tuberculosis.

In the developing world, however, the position is very different, for today tuberculosis remains a major burden on the health of these lands, with an annual risk of infection ten times higher than that in the developed countries, and tragically these rates do not seem to be falling rapidly (Fig. 60). In England and Wales in 1978–9, some 70% of all the 7000 newly notified cases of tuberculosis had pulmonary tuberculosis, and about one-third of these were infectious with acid fast-bacilli seen in their sputum smear. Patients originating ethnically from India, Pakistan and Bangladesh had the highest rate of infection, particularly of non-respiratory tuberculosis. In the general population those most at risk of developing clinical tuberculosis include very young children and *immune suppressed patients* (see Chapters 2 and 8).

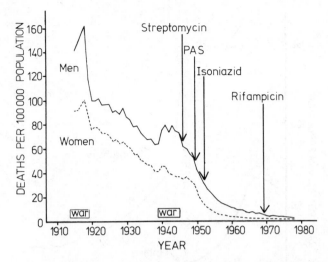

*Fig. 58.*    Annual death rate for tuberculosis (England and Wales) from 1915 to 1978, showing the rise during each World War, but nonetheless a steady fall, greatly accelerated by classical chemotherapy (streptomycin, PAS and isoniazid)

## Pathogenesis and pathology

Infection spreads principally by inhalation of *Mycobacterium tuberculosis* carried on droplet nuclei of 1–10 μm diameter, which are derived from an untreated patient with open (smear-positive) pulmonary tuberculosis. Bovine milk-borne tuberculosis is almost eliminated today in developed countries and unboiled cow's milk is not often drunk in undeveloped countries. Deposit of droplet nuclei containing *M. tuberculosis* in the alveoli of a previously uninfected human provokes production of an exudate containing polymorphs which ingest some bacilli. These polymorphs are speedily followed by alveolar macrophages and blood monocytes which phagocytose both free bacilli and the polymorph-containing bacilli, and so become transformed into *epithelioid cells* lying in the centre of the granulomatous lesions known as the *primary tubercle*, surrounded by a cuff of lymphocytes and later fibroblasts (Fig. 61). Within three to eight weeks the patient develops *hypersensitivity* to tubercular protein, as shown by a positive tuberculin skin test. T lymphocytes are then sensitized to release lymphokines which activate macrophages, so enhancing their power of bacterial killing, and at this time *caseation* or necrosis of the epithelioid cells occurs in the centre of the tubercle.

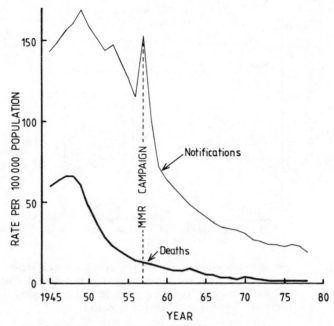

*Fig. 59.*    Notifications and death rates from tuberculosis in Scotland from 1945 to 1978. The rate has fallen little in recent years and the disease has not been irradicated

Some of these epithelioid cells become *multinucleate giant cells*. The lymphatic glands draining this lesion may show similar involvement, the combination together being termed the primary complex.

In many this primary lesion heals completely, sometimes with calcification, but leaves the positive skin test to tuberculin as the only evidence of this primary infection. Rarely the primary complex leads on to progressive disease, which may take the form of:

1.  Haematogenous spread, with *miliary tuberculosis* and *tuberculous meningitis*, most frequently within one year of the primary infection.

2.  Chronic haematogenous spread to *bone or joints* within three to five years of the primary infection, or to the genitourinary tract, where lesions may not develop for five to 15 years after the primary infection.

3.  *Tuberculous pleural effusion*, usually within one year.

4.  Bronchial involvement, either due to local bronchial obstruction by an enlarged tuberculous hilar gland or from an inflammatory exudate which may rarely progress to tuberculous caseous bronchopneumonia. These bronchial complications occur within six to nine months of the primary infection.

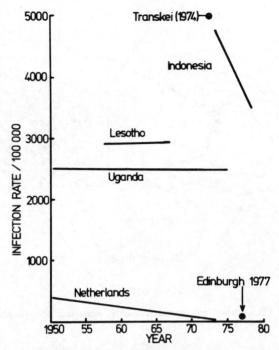

*Fig. 60.*    Annual risk of tuberculous infection in some different countries in the world, between 1950 and 1978. Data from the International Union Against Tuberculosis, 1978

5. Tubercle bacilli spread to the lungs as part of a haematogenous spread, but there remain dormant, and may cause post-primary tuberculosis in later life.

*Erythema nodosum* is characterized by raised tender purplish red swellings on the front of the calves and rarely on the elbows, particularly in young women, and can be an index of tuberculous hypersensitivity following a primary infection. A similar hyper-sensitivity reaction to tuberculin is *phlyctenular conjunctivitis*.

# Primary tuberculosis

## Clinical features

Primary tuberculous infection in adults is usually asymptomatic. It is, of course, indicated by the development of a positive tuberculin skin test. Radiological evidence of the primary focus develops in under one-third of cases, the glandular component of this being more likely to be detected in children. The uncomplicated primary lesion rarely causes

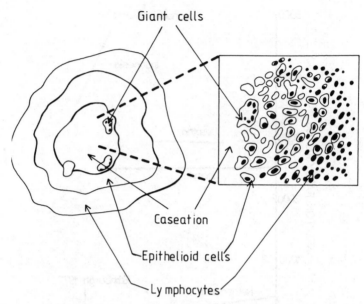

*Fig. 61*    The pathology of tuberculosis, showing the pattern of the tubercle, and cellular constituents

symptoms in children, but may produce fever, failure to gain weight, anorexia, lethargy and dyspnoea; cough is not usually prominent. Vague ill health in a child in contact with a known case of tuberculosis should lead to tuberculin skin testing. If the result remains negative on two occasions separated by six weeks, tuberculosis is very unlikely to be the cause of any illness. An apparent pneumonic shadow on the chest radiograph, which does not clear with antibiotics within 14 days, is suggestive of tuberculosis in a child, even if the glandular component of the primary complex is not prominent, but again the diagnosis would be confirmed by a positive tuberculin test.

### The tuberculin test

The intradermal injection of a purified protein derivative (PPD) of cultured tubercle bacilli produces a cell-mediated immune reaction (Type IV) with induration and erythema of the skin at the site of injection. In the *Mantoux* test 0.1 ml of old tuberculin is injected *intradermally*, the test being read at 48–72 hours, when a positive result is indicated by an area of induration of at least 6 mm in diameter (Fig. 62). When hypersensitivity may be marked, as in erythema nodosum or with a suspected tuberculous pleural effusion or phlyctenular conjunctivitis, 1:10 000 solution is used; if the response is

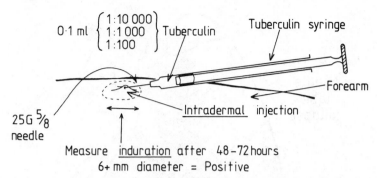

<figure>
0.1 ml { 1:10 000 / 1:1 000 / 1:100 } Tuberculin — Tuberculin syringe

— Forearm

Intradermal injection

25G ⅝ needle

Measure induration after 48-72 hours
6+ mm diameter = Positive
</figure>

*Fig. 62.*   The Mantoux test, whereby 0.1 ml of a dilution of old tuberculin injected *intradermally*, so as to raise a bleb within the skin, causes an induration of at least 6 mm diameter, read at 48–72 hours, as a positive response

negative, this is followed by 1:1000 and then 1:100 solution if the response to 1:1000 is negative. The *Heaf* test uses a six-point multiple puncture 'gun', which following sterilization is applied to the skin which has previously been swabbed with PPD in a strength of 2 mg/ml; the 'gun' is then triggered, so causing the punctures to penetrate 1–2 mm below the skin surface. The test is read at three to five days, a Grade III reaction (where the six separate papules form a ring with a filled centre) being definitely positive. The *Tine* test uses four 2 mm long prongs smeared with sterilized old tuberculin which is pressed into the skin, but its validity is under question at present.

Other diagnostic approaches in primary tuberculosis include attempts to culture bacilli from gastric washings, or laryngeal swabs, these being mainly indicated if there is a chance that the child has been infected with drug-resistant bacilli.

With the efficacy and safety of modern chemotherapy based on rifampicin and isoniazid (see later), most authorities recommend treatment of a child in whom the tuberculin tests converts from negative to positive, and all agree that the presence of a primary lesion demonstrated radiologically is a definite indication for treatment.

## Complications

Homogeneous opacities, often of lobar distribution (*epituberculosis*), can be due to: (1) collapse from pressure of a large tuberculous gland on a bronchus or tuberculous bronchostenosis, both involving the middle lobe (Fig. 63); (2) inflammatory exudates within the lobe due to the hypersensitivity phenomenon; or (3) a caseous pneumonia.

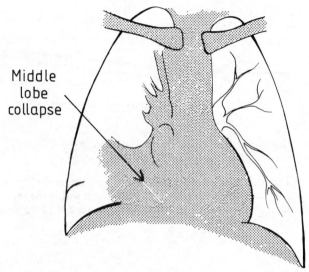

Middle
lobe
collapse

*Fig. 63.*    Primary tuberculosis causing middle lobe collapse and consolidation in a child

Crepitations in diminished movement are common and the symptoms may be those of otherwise uncomplicated primary tuberculosis. Bronchiectasis may be a late complication of such lesions.

*Erythema nodosum* can be evidence of tuberculous hypersensitivity, but the commonest cause in Britain is probably sarcoidosis, usually associated with bilateral lymphadenopathy. Other causes of erythema nodosum include drug reactions (sulphonamides, including cotrimoxazole), streptococcal infections, and, on a world-wide scale, leprosy. Fever and pains in the wrists and large joints may be associated, as is a high ESR.

*Phlyctenular conjunctivitis*, with photophobia, pain and reddening of the eyes, is another manifestation of tuberculous hypersensitivity. A small 1–2 mm bleb at the limbus with a leash of vessels running to it is characteristic. Hydrocortisone drops rapidly relieve the symptoms, but the tuberculosis causing the lesion also requires treatment.

A *pleural effusion*, which may be large, characteristically shows a clear fluid with a predominance of lymphocytes and this is common in primary tuberculosis arising after puberty. Pleural biopsy may yield typical tubercles, but the organism is rarely seen in smears of the pleural fluid, although a positive culture is most likely if a large volume of the fluid is sent to the laboratory.

The *haematogenous spread of tuberculosis* is always a risk in primary infection, particularly in children.

*Miliary tuberculosis*, in which multiple tubercles composed of

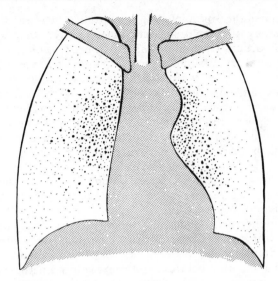

*Fig. 64.*    Sketch of chest radiograph in miliary tuberculosis, showing the diffuse snowstorm pattern, maximal at the hilar regions, but spreading throughout both lung fields. In any case, the opacities are usually of the same size, but may be small, as here, or larger, up to 10 mm in diameter

epithelioid cells, giant cells and a cuff of lymphocytes are widely distributed throughout the body, nearly always including the lungs, is the major hazard, for this can lead to *tuberculous meningitis*, which was invariably fatal before the introduction of chemotherapy.

Measles and whooping cough are recognized precipitants of miliary tuberculosis, which usually presents as a gradual onset of ill health, with loss of weight and fever. Hepatosplenomegaly is present in about 30% of cases, and chest signs are late, often consisting of no more than widespread fine crepitations. *Choroidal tubercles* occur in up to 35% of acute cases and are pathognomic of miliary tuberculosis, but do not necessarily indicate that tuberculous meningitis is complicating the miliary spread. They appear in the fundi as honey-coloured roughly circular lesions about one-quarter of the diameter of the optic disc and are so important diagnostically that a thorough search under a general anaesthetic may be justified in a child who cannot cooperate.

The chest radiograph in miliary tuberculosis classically shows multiple small discrete opacities, varying in any one case from 1–2 mm up to 5–10 mm in diameter (Fig. 64). In a febrile child, pneumonia due to mycoplasma or respiratory syncytical virus (RSV) can give similar appearances, but the white blood count is usually normal in miliary tuberculosis, and such pneumonic opacities will clear within two weeks of chemotherapy (including tetracycline), whereas shadowing due to miliary tuberculosis clears more slowly, even with anti-tuberculosis drugs, which should *always* be used in any case of doubt. In the *adult* miliary tuberculosis may present as pyrexia of unknown origin (*cryptic miliary tuberculosis*). *Blood dyscrasias* are then not infrequent and the diagnosis may only be proved by bone marrow or liver biopsy, showing miliary tubercles, with or without acid-fast bacilli. A clinical response within one or two weeks of starting treatment with specific antituberculous drugs, such as isoniazid and ethambutol, may be the only alternative way of proving the diagnosis, as in the elderly the tuberculin skin test may be only weakly positive in cryptic miliary tuberculosis. Reactivation of previous tuberculous infection can occur in immunosuppressed patients, as for example in those receiving corticosteroids.

The complications of miliary tuberculosis include *tuberculous meningitis*, which may only be indicated by behavioural abnormalities, headache, vomiting and vague ill health, or an isolated fit, but can proceed to alternating delirium and coma with numerous localizing signs, often involving cranial nerves. The CSF is crystal clear at the outset of miliary tuberculosis and although polymorphs may be the predominant cells within the first 48 hours, lymphocytes thereafter predominate. Glucose concentration of CSF is characteristically much lower than that in simultaneously taken serum, but the protein concentration is high. Acid-fast bacilli may be found only on careful search of the characteristic 'spider's web' clot forming in the CSF. A normal CSF does not exclude tuberculous meningitis and the examination should be repeated 24 hours later if the clinical diagnosis remains a possibility.

Antituberculous chemotherapy can be life-saving in tuberculous meningitis, but should include four antituberculous drugs, as rifampicin, 10 mg/kg in adults and up to 20 mg/kg in children, per day; isoniazid, 10–12 mg/kg daily given intramuscularly or intravenously; pyrazinamide 30 mg/kg to a maximum of 2.5 g daily; and streptomycin 1.0 g daily, or 0.75 g daily if the patient is aged over 45 years, by intramuscular injection. Pyridoxine 50 mg daily by mouth is also given, to prevent the risk of peripheral neuropathy from this high dose of isoniazid, and corticosteroids (30 mg/day prednisolone orally), to prevent the develop of adhesions leading to obstructive hydrocephalus. Hypokalaemia developing during the course of treatment can be a dangerous complication and is particularly liable to occur in elderly women.

# Post-primary pulmonary tuberculosis

This is the most common form of tuberculosis and these cases form the main source of infection within the community. The primary lesion can progress, despite the state of hypersensitivity, and this is most likely to occur if the primary infection occurs after puberty. However, in most subjects the cell-mediated immune process prevents the development of progressive post-primary tuberculosis, but some authorities believe that a decline in T cell function with age may be responsible for reactivation of such previously quiescent infection, but this matter is controversial. The lymphatics from the primary focus drain into the thoracic duct, so leading to haematogenous spread to the lungs. The predilection for such infection to localize in the lung apices is thought to result from the high $Po_2$ of that part of the lungs, resulting from the high apical ventilation–perfusion ratio in the upright posture. Reinfection must overcome the protection afforded by tuberculin hypersensitivity and this is therefore probably an uncommon cause of post-primary pulmonary tuberculosis.

Pathologically the tuberculous granuloma is the hallmark of post-primary tuberculosis, tubercles developing at the periphery of a lesion whose centre is occupied by necrotic caseous tissue, which may become liquified and coughed out, so forming the tuberculous cavity. The tubercle, with central epithelioid cells and Langhan's giant cells abutting on to areas of caseation, is surrounded by a cuff of lymphocytes and then fibroblasts (see Fig. 61). The tubercle heals by fibrosis with local contracture. Calcification is a less common end result than in the primary tuberculous lesion, but calcified lesions can still yield viable tubercle bacilli. Chemotherapy accelerates the fibrosis, the cavities shrinking and many eventually closing.

## Clinical features

Symptoms are often initially non-specific with weakness and tiredness, associated with anorexia and weight loss, whereas persistent cough, the commonest respiratory symptom, may only be elicited after direct questioning. There can be no symptoms, despite active smear positive disease. Haemoptysis is characteristic and the direct question 'Have you ever coughed-up blood?' should always be included in history-taking. Night sweats, which may drench the pyjamas, are a classical symptom, but today relatively uncommon. Irritability, sleeplessness and poor concentration may also be symptoms of tuberculous toxaemia, but clearly have many other potential causes. Dyspepsia and amenorrhoea are recognized features. Tuberculosis can be a cause of acute pneumonia, when acid-fast bacilli are found in the sputum smear.

On examination tachycardia may be related to the fever. Finger-clubbing is unusual in early cases, unless the disease is very pronounced. Crepitations after cough over the apices may be the only physical sign, but it is today rare to detect the classical signs of the

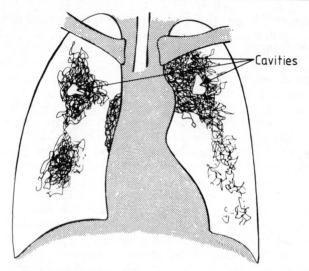

Cavities

*Fig. 65.*    Sketch of chest radiograph showing bilateral upper lobe cavitated lesions in a case of active post-primary pulmonary tuberculosis, with a positive smear

cavity with amphoric breathing and a cracked-pot percussion note. Signs of consolidation may be present in tuberculous pneumonia.

The *chest radiograph* is the major means of determining the anatomical location and extent of the disease, but the diagnosis can only be proven bacteriologically. The disease characteristically appears as opacities in the upper lobes, or in the apex of the lower lobes, usually showing as patchy shadows with characteristic cavities (Fig. 65) which may be clearly seen only on tomography. The lesions are usually bilateral, but not symmetrical. The shadows persist despite treatment with antibacterial non-antituberculous antibiotics. Post-primary tuberculosis is rarely seen only in the anterior segment of an upper lobe, the apical and posterior segments being more usually involved, with a slight predominance to disease in the right lung. Although such patchy cavitated apical lesions are characteristic, there are a wide variety of appearances. Soft shadows may suggest a pneumonic process, tuberculosis being suspected only when these do not resolve with time; whereas linear opacities, with distortion of mediastinal structures due to hilar gland enlargement, are rarely prominent in post-primary tuberculosis in Europeans, but are a well recognized presentation in Asian and African patients.

A normal chest radiograph probably excludes pulmonary tuberculosis, but even experts can miss abnormalities on single readings. In a comprehensive international study, 5% of patients with sputum smear-positive tuberculosis were reported as having a normal chest radiograph and in 24% of such cases the radiograph was interpreted as indicating that no clinical action was needed!

*Bacteriological examination of sputum* is thus imperative to establish the diagnosis firmly, but acid-fast bacilli are still identified by smear or culture in only 60% of those currently being notified as suffering from tuberculosis in the United Kingdom. A sputum smear will probably be regarded as positive if it contains 100 000 acid-fast bacilli per millilitre. Smear examination is the preferred method of case finding in the developing countries, as it is more precise, clinically relevant and less costly than radiological surveys. Patients with positive sputum smears are infectious, at least until they start treatment. Furthermore, without treatment most smear-positive patients will die of tuberculosis. Sputum culture, which is clearly more sensitive than direct examination of sputum smears, only gives results in four to eight weeks, three specimens of sputum usually being examined by either smear or culture.

Gastric lavage, laryngeal swab or, rarely, bronchial lavage may also yield positive smears or cultures. In case finding, induced coughing with production of sputum following inhalation of nebulized saline for 15 minutes, has been found to be of value in rural Africa.

# Treatment

Chemotherapy, starting with Waksman's discovery of streptomycin in 1941, has revolutionized the outlook for the patient with tuberculosis, the condition today being curable. Early relapse following the use of single drug chemotherapy soon led to the evolution of triple drug regimens, *classical chemotherapy* consisting of 18 months of treatment with streptomycin, isoniazid and *para*-aminosalicyclic acid (PAS). Current *standard chemotherapy* uses oral rifampicin (450 mg/day for those under 50 kg body weight; 600 mg/day for those over 50 kg body weight), isoniazid (300 mg/day) and ethambutol (15 mg/kg/day) for two months, all given once daily before breakfast on an empty stomach. This is then followed by a continuation of rifampicin and isoniazid in the above doses for a further seven months, giving a total treatment duration of nine months. Combination capsules contain rifampicin with isoniazid, providing 150 mg rifampicin with 100 mg isoniazid, or 300 mg rifampicin with 150 mg isoniazid. This regimen has proved to be highly effective for treatment of tuberculosis in the United Kingdom.

Antituberculous drug regimens succeed by two actions: bactericidal (killing dividing bacilli), where isoniazid and rifampicin are particularly active, and sterilization, killing persistent bacilli which are not dividing, which thus have a very low metabolic rate. Isoniazid with pyrazinamide is a potent sterilizing combination and rifampicin also has activity in this sterilizing role. Newer regimens of shorter course chemotherapy are being actively pursued, notably by the British Medical Research Council, in trials in Singapore, Hong Kong and Kenya and in the United Kingdom by the British Thoracic Association. A six-month regimen, starting with two months of daily streptomycin, isoniazid, rifampicin and pyrazinamide, followed by a further four months of rifampicin and isoniazid, has achieved considerable success in Singapore and is being evaluated elsewhere. However, these regimens are currently experimental, and the *recommended regimen remains the standard nine months of rifampicin with ioniazid, with the addition of ethambutol for the first two months.*

## Side effects of antituberculous drugs

*Rifampicin* usually causes the urine to become orange-red and patients should be warned of this. Anorexia, nausea and vomiting may occur at the start of treatment. The liver enzymes (aspartate aminotransaminase and isocitrate dehydrogenase) often rise temporarily in the first week of treatment, thereafter returning to normal despite continuation of rifampicin. Clinical hepatitis with jaundice probably occurs in less than 1% of cases treated with rifampicin. Thrombocytopenic purpura is a rare but recognized complication of rifampicin and requires permanent withdrawal of the drug. Regimens using intermittent rifampicin can produce a 'flu-like' illness with fever, chills, bone pains and malaise, which starts after three to six months of treatment, but only when rifampicin is given once or twice a week. This may be associated with circulating antibodies to rifampicin. Rifampicin *induces liver enzymes which metabolize* some drugs, so necessitating adjustment of the dose of oral anticoagulants, digoxin and sulphonylureas. The action of oral contraceptives is similarly impaired, and an alternative means of contraception should be used whilst the patient is on rifampicin treatment. Cortisol metabolism is enhanced and steroid doses (e.g. for Addison's disease or immunosuppression) must be increased.

The patient's compliance with drug therapy is the major remaining problem in the treatment of tuberculosis, and this can be checked by noting the red colour in the urine, which is clearly shown by extraction of urine with butanol.

*Isoniazid* in the dose of up to 300 mg daily rarely causes side effects. Hypersensitivity, with fever, drug rash and lymphadenopathy, is recognized. Peripheral neuropathy can occur with higher doses, but can be prevented by giving pyridoxine (10 mg) along with isoniazid.

*Ethambutol* can cause retrobulbar neuritis. This is very rare unless the dose of 15 mg/kg/day is exceeded. The eye changes revert on withdrawing the drug. Patients receiving ethambutol should be asked to report any visual disturbances immediately.

*Pyrazinamide* can cause hepatitis, usually preceded by anorexia, nausea and vomiting. A gouty arthropathy, with raised levels of uric acid, responding to allopurinol, is an uncommon but recognized side effect.

## Other antituberculosis drugs

Classical chemotherapy (streptomycin, *para*-aminosalicylic acid and isoniazid for 18 months) has now been replaced by rifampicin-based regimens in developed countries, but classical chemotherapy is still much cheaper and thus still in use in the developing world. Streptomycin in this regimen is often given three times weekly, as, of course, the drug must be given by intramuscular injection. Other drugs (second line or reserve drugs) are used for treatment if the organisms are known to be resistant to standard chemotherapeutic agents. These reserve drugs include ethionamide, cycloserine, capreomycin and viomycin, but are all less active than standard chemotherapeutic agents and have more severe side effects.

*Corticosteroids* are used to suppress an intense cell-mediated immune reaction to tuberculoprotein, but clearly this is safe only if the patient is already receiving an effective antituberculous regimen. Corticosteroids are therefore used in the treatment of tuberculous meningitis, pericarditis, peritonitis and genitourinary tuberculosis. In tuberculous pleural effusions corticosteroids can probably speed the rate of reabsorption of the exudate. As rifampicin induces hepatic corticosteroid metabolism, a dose of 40–60 mg/day is used, reducing over two or three weeks, to be discontinued in six weeks as the inflammatory response subsides.

## Cost of antituberculosis drugs

Tuberculosis remains a major problem in the developing world, where the cost of the regimen may be critical. In 1976 the standard chemotherapeutic regimen (rifampicin, isoniazid for nine months, with ethambutol for the first two months) cost £250 in Britain, 90% of this being for the rifampicin. This regimen costs two and a half times less in Algeria, which may be representative of a developing country. Conversely, streptomycin, isoniazid and pyrazinamide, given on a thrice weekly basis, had a success rate of 94% over a nine-month course, and cost only £40 in 1978 in Hong Kong, but some £25 in Algeria. However, a rational choice of treatment regimens should include the costs of supervision of therapy, of retreating patients who fail to respond and of the cases of drug toxicity induced by the treatment.

*Primary drug resistance*, nearly always to either streptomycin or isoniazid, was present in about 8% of the cases in the United Kingdom which originated from the Indian Subcontinent in 1978–9. However, this problem was only seen in under 2% of other UK cases at the same time.

# Prevention

Cure of patients who cough out tubercule bacilli, particularly the patient with post-primary cavitated pulmonary disease, must be the primary aim. After starting a modern effective antituberculous drug regimen, such patients rapidly become non-infectious, although they may still excrete non-viable bacilli for some months. Thus, isolation of the patient is no longer required. Increasing the resistance of the host to infection is the aim of *BCG vaccination*. BCG (bacille Calmette–Guérin) induces cell-mediated immunity, dependent on T cells, to tuberculoprotein. This is currently offered routinely in the UK to tuberculin-negative 12–13-year-old school children, and has been proved to reduce the risk of disseminated tuberculosis following primary infection by 70% for at least 10 years thereafter. BCG is also used to protect tuberculin-negative contacts, including the infants of tuberculous mothers. However, a recent careful trial of BCG in South India showed that it failed to confer protective effects in that specific population. In developed countries, careful tracing of contacts of newly notified cases of tuberculosis is a very important method of detecting new cases that need treatment. Such contact examination should be concentrated upon those who are exposed to smear-positive patients.

*Chemoprophylaxis* aims to prevent infection in those particularly at risk, as in a breast-fed baby of a tuberculous mother, where the baby may be given BCG (using an isoniazid-resistant strain of organism), combined with treatment with isoniazid alone in a dose of 5 mg/kg. Chemopropylaxis is also used to prevent the development of the disease in those who are known to have been infected, e.g. patients who have shown a conversion of a tuberculin skin test from negative to positive, in strongly tuberculin-positive young contacts, and in tuberculin-positive patients who are to start immunosuppresive therapy (see Chapter 8).

## Further reading

FOX, W. (1980) Short course chemotherapy for tuberculosis. In *Recent Advances in Respiratory Medicine II*, ed. D. C. Flenley. Edinburgh: Churchill Livingstone.

KEERS, R. Y. (1978) *Pulmonary Tuberculosis: A Journey Down the Centuries*. London: Baillière Tindall.

MEDICAL RESEARCH COUNCIL TUBERCULOSIS AND CHEST DISEASES UNIT (1980) National survey of tuberculosis notifications in England and Wales 1978-9. *Br. med. J.*, **2**, 895-898.

STYLBO, K. (1980) Recent advances in epidemiological research in tuberculosis. *Adv. Tuberc. Res.*, **20**, 1-63.

TOMEN, K. (1979) *Tuberculosis: Case Finding and Chemotherapy; Questions and Answers*. Geneva: World Health Organization.

WOLINSKY, E. (1979) Nontuberculous myobacteria and associated diseases. *Am. Rev. resp. Dis.*, **119**, 107-159.

# 14

# Pulmonary Tumours

Nearly all tumours of the lungs are malignant, bronchial carcinoma being by far the most frequent, tumours of lesser malignancy (carcinoid and cylindroma) being much less common, and the benign connective tissue neoplasm, or hamartoma, relatively rare.

## Bronchial carcinoma

### Epidemiology

Bronchial carcinoma is now the commonest cause of death from malignant disease in men in the Western hemisphere and is second only to that from breast cancer in women. This unenviable position has only recently been achieved and in most countries the death rate from lung cancer is still increasing, particularly in women (Fig. 66). The death rate is higher in the United Kingdom than in the USA, that in Scotland being the highest in the world. Most cases occur in men over 50 years of age and the disease is uncommon under age 30.

In 1952 Doll and Bradford Hill clearly showed that more patients with bronchial carcinoma than control patients were smokers and this result has been confirmed throughout the world, in both retrospective and prospective studies. People whose religion precludes smoking, such as Seventh Day Adventists in the USA and Parsi Indians in Bombay, have very low death rates from lung cancer. Furthermore, the risk rises with the number of cigarettes smoked and falls as the years progress after giving up the habit. Nearly all accept that cigarette smoking causes lung cancer, despite the undoubted difficulty of producing a human type of bronchial carcinoma from exposure of animals to cigarette tar. It strains belief to accept that cigarette smoking (an acquired habit) and susceptibility to bronchial carcinoma both arise from the same genetic make-up. However, the cigarette that is smoked has changed with the introduction of filter tips, with a gradual trend to lower yields of tar, today's very low tar cigarettes having ventilated filters in which the smoke inhaled is diluted by air drawn in through the filter. However, these very low tar- and nicotine-

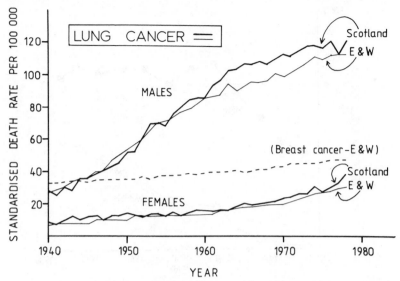

*Fig. 66.* Standardized death rates per 100 000 of population from lung cancer and breast cancer in Scotland and England and Wales

yielding cigarettes have only a small fraction of the total market and the epidemiological evidence seems clearly to indicate that there is *no safe cigarette* (Figs 66, 67).

The 1200 separate chemical substances in tobacco smoke include many known carcinogens, including 3,4-benzpyrene and polonium-210. The recent identification of individuals in whom *aryl hydrocarbon hydroxylase (AHH)* on cell surfaces can be readily induced by exposure to carcinogens in cigarette smoke, in contrast to other individuals in whom this enzyme cannot be so readily induced, has led to the demonstration that such easily inducible AHH subjects are more frequently found amongst lung cancer patients. This would imply that such people may be particularly at risk of developing lung cancer if they smoke, but this work remains to be confirmed.

*Occupational hazards* leading to an increased risk of lung cancer are clearly recognized, but are much less important to the individual than is cigarette smoking. Asbestos exposure interacts with cigarette smoking to increase the risk of lung cancer greatly, in addition to the specific risks of developing pleural mesothelioma (see Chapter 17), and it has long been known that exposure to radio-active materials, as in uranium miners, also increases the risk of lung cancer. Nickel ore, chloromethyl methyl ether (in ion-exchange resins), bichromates, haematite and industrial arsenic exposure are also recognized risk factors.

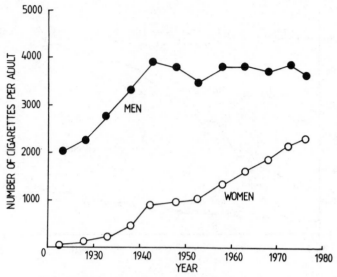

*Fig. 67.*    Cigarette consumption in the UK population over 15 years of age,
showing that although this may have reached a plateau in men, it
is still rising in women. Compare this with the death rates from
lung cancer in Fig. 66 (*From N. J. Wald (1976) Lancet, 1, 136*)

## Pathology and pathogenesis

Bronchial carcinoma probably starts in the basal cells of the respiratory epithelium, which lie between the columnar epithelial and
goblet cells and the basement membrane. Smoking causes these cells to
increase in number and their nuclei to become atypical and hyperchro-
matic, leading to squamous metaplasia and replacement locally of the
ciliated cells. Mitoses then develop in the basal cell layer, leading to
carcinoma-in-situ. Invasion is indicated by penetration of the basement membrane. Clinical presentation and response to therapy of the
four characteristic pathological types of bronchial carcinoma are so
different that it is now realized that identification of the cell type is
highly desirable in order to plan a rational programme of treatment.

*Squamous carcinoma (epidermoid carcinoma)* is the commonest cell
type, with an incidence varying from 40 to 70% of all cases, depending
upon the source of the material (autopsy, surgical resection, bronchial
biopsy, etc.). On light microscopy typical squamous cell tumours show
intracellular bridges, with formation of cell nests where squamous
cells are arranged in a polarised or whorl pattern (Fig. 68A). Poorly
differentiated squamous cell carcinomas merge histologically with the
anaplastic or poorly differentiated large cell carcinomas. Squamous
cancer may arise either centrally, where the tumour often obstructs a

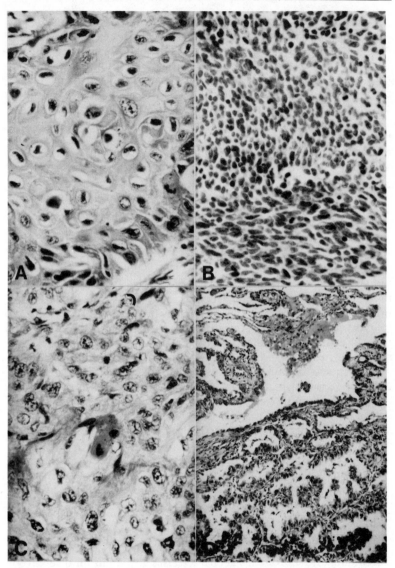

*Fig. 68.*    Histological appearances of the four different types of bronchial carcinoma. A, Squamous carcinoma, B, Small (oat) cell carcinoma, C, Large cell carcinoma, D. Adenocarcinoma

major bronchus, or peripherally. Cavitation is relatively common in squamous carcinoma and the tumours are slow-growing, but do *not* respond to currently available chemotherapy. However, most of these tumours are initially radiosensitive.

*Anaplastic carcinoma* can present as three different types:

1. *Small round cell (oat cell) carcinoma*, with cells showing little cytoplasm, are usually monotonously similar on histological section (Fig. 68B). These tumours, which may account for up to 20–30% of all bronchial carcinoma cases, are highly malignant and many regard them as being disseminated throughout the body from the time of diagnosis. They rarely arise peripherally and seldom cavitate within the lungs, but can occlude bronchi. Electron microscopy has suggested that these tumours (which are particularly associated with ectopic hormone production; see later) may originate from cells of the APUD system, as shown by the presence of electron dense neurosecretory granules.

2. *Large cell carcinoma*, where cells are the same size as those of squamous cell tumours, but do not show the characteristic whorled or nest-like appearance (Fig. 68C), accounts for 10–15% of bronchial carcinoma.

3. *Adenocarcinoma*, which characteristically arises in the periphery of the lungs, presenting as a capillary or solid alveolar form, these tumours often producing mucus (Fig. 68D). Although previously thought to be relatively rare, accounting for some 10% of all cases of bronchial carcinoma, this type of cancer *appears to be becoming more frequent*, at least in North America, where some have claimed that it is now the commonest of all types of bronchial carcinoma. However, this may in part reflect a fashion in pathological diagnosis. This tumour is more frequent in women and appears to be the commonest type of cancer to arise in scars in the lung, particularly those which have resulted from pulmonary infarcts in the upper lobes. The tumour spreads somewhat less rapidly than oat cell cancer, but is also less sensitive to modern chemotherapy. Brain metastases are particularly common.

*Alveolar cell carcinoma* is rare and derives from the alveolar type II cell. It is not related to smoking. It is easily confused with metastases from adenocarcinomata elsewhere in the body, as it often presents with diffuse nodulation involving *both lungs*.

## Clinical features

Carcinoma of the bronchus is characteristically silent until relatively late in its life cycle, which may be on average some 10 years after the initial malignant cellular change, which, of course, occurs long before the tumour is detected. Symptoms and signs tend to present in three patterns.

The *primary tumour* causes increasing cough as the commonest presenting feature, but most smokers regard a morning cough as normal. *Haemoptysis* is of outstanding importance. It is usually small, may be repeated and can be hidden unless the direct question is asked

'Have you ever coughed up blood?'. Haemoptysis always needs to be taken seriously and *never* merely dismissed as 'a small blood vessel bursting at the back of the throat'! Other common causes of haemoptysis include tuberculosis, pneumonia, pulmonary infarction, bronchiectasis and mitral stenosis. Every patient with haemoptysis should be suspected to be suffering from lung cancer and, after careful clinical examination, should always have at least one chest radiograph and sputum examination for *M. tuberculosis*.

*Breathlessness*, which as with other conditions is nearly always worse on exertion, is rarely a presenting feature of lung cancer, but can indicate the development of a complication such as a pleural effusion or bronchial obstruction with collapse of the lung behind the obstruction.

*Chest pain*, which may be of dull boring character, not typical of pleuritic or anginal pain, can be a presenting feature of bronchial carcinoma, and some consider it to indicate mediastinal gland involvement. Pleuritic pain in bronchial carcinoma suggests pneumonic complications such as pneumonia behind a blocked bronchus, or direct invasion of the pleura by the tumour.

*Pneumonia*, particularly in a *man* who smokes and is over 50 years of age, should always raise the possibility of an underlying lung cancer, particularly if the pneumonia is slow to clear. 'Infection behind the block' from a centrally placed bronchial carcinoma is very common. Localized wheeze may also raise the suspicion of partial obstruction of a lobar bronchus by bronchial carcinoma.

*Symptoms from local spread* can include *hoarseness of the voice* due to involvement of the recurrent laryngeal nerve, this being more frequent in tumours involving the left mediastinal nodes. Hoarseness which persists for longer than three weeks always requires investigation, but, of course, a neoplasm of the vocal cords or of the larynx is also a possibility. *Stridor*, a musical note during expiration, implies a lesion involving the main bronchi or trachea, which may arise either from a tumour in the airway wall or from external compression by enlarged glands involved in metastases.

*Superior vena caval obstruction* often presents as a characteristic picture with headache, suffusion of the face and conjunctivae, fullness of the neck and even oedema of the hands on the affected side. The external jugular veins are engorged and the other veins over the hemithorax are dilated. The symptoms include dysphagia and stridor and result from tumour compressing the great veins draining from the head and arm.

A *superior sulcus (Pancoast) tumour* commonly erodes the neck of the first rib (or other upper ribs) and involves the brachial plexus and the cervical sympathetic nerves. The patient may therefore complain of pain in the inner aspect of the arm (T1 dermatome) and may have a *Horner's syndrome* (small pupil, partial ptosis, enophthalmus and lack of thermal sweating all on that side of the face) and wasting of the small muscles of the hand on the affected side. This tumour is nearly always a squamous carcinoma and is unusual in that radiotherapy *before* operative removal has been shown to prolong survival.

Invasion of the *pericardium* and heart, causing arrhythmias including heart block with pericardial pain and ST elevation on the ECG, with a blood-stained pericardial effusion, can be fatal from cardiac tamponade.

A *pleural effusion* from which metastatic cells may be obtained on pleural biopsy, or more rarely from examination of the pleural fluid, is well recognized as a presenting feature of bronchial carcinoma. Such an effusion will usually be *blood-stained*, and must be therefore differentiated from an effusion due to pulmonary infarction (see Chapter 20).

*Distant spread* by metastases most frequently occurs to the brain, liver, bone and suprarenals. Brain metastases may present as behaviour disorders or as the classical signs of raised intracranial pressure with papilloedema, vomiting and bradycardia, or of epilepsy of recent onset. Thus any adult male smoker presenting with epilepsy of recent onset should always have a chest radiograph. Pain from bony metastases may be a presenting feature, as in the back pain from vertebral collapse or a pathological fracture in a long bone. Addison's disease can result from bilateral suprarenal gland metastases, but hyperpigmentation can also arise from production of melanocyte-stimulating hormone (MSH), particularly by an oat cell bronchial carcinoma. Enlargement of the liver and/or palpable supraclavicular nodes may occasionally be the presenting feature and these should always be sought on examination. Weight loss, tiredness and anorexia, although frequently mentioned as presenting features of bronchial carcinoma, are usually associated with at least some respiratory symptoms.

## Examination

*Clubbing of the fingers* is common, possibly more so with oat cell cancer, and best recognized by in-filling of the angle between the normal nail and nail bed (see Chapter 5). It may appear first in the index fingers. The nail bed may be abnormally fluctuant, but absence of this sign, which is a subjective judgement made by the physician, should never lead the unwary to dismiss obvious clubbing as of no significance. Other causes of clubbing (see Chapter 5) should be included and one should always beware of accepting a patient's statement that 'his fingers have always been like that', or 'all my family have fingers like that', *without* checking this personally.

In the chest atelectasis (collapse) is the commonest sign of lung cancer as shown by diminished movement, mediastinal shift (as shown by the apex beat position and position of the trachea), dullness to

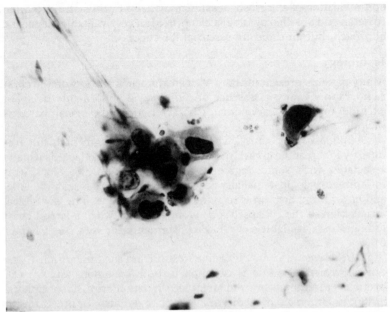

*Fig. 69.*  Photomicrograph of malignant cells in sputum, derived from a squamous carcinoma of the bronchus

percussion and reduced breath sounds over the affected zone. Bronchial breathing will be heard over an apical collapsed lobe, irrespective of whether the major bronchus is occluded by bronchial carcinoma, but over a lower lobe bronchial breathing is rare when collapse arises from bronchial carcinoma, as this sign implies that the lower lobe bronchus is patent so conducting the sounds from the trachea and larynx, as in the consolidation of lobar pneumonia.

The physical signs of any complicating pneumonia, pleural effusion or pericardial involvement may be present. Diaphragmatic palsy may be revealed by basal dullness, which can be confused with pleural effusion, but is more usually only confirmed by screening of diaphragmatic movement. Cervical lymph nodes, particularly the scalene nodes, should be carefully palpated, as should the liver for evidence of enlargement from metastases.

### Sputum cytology

Identification of malignant cells in sputum (Fig. 69) can yield proof of the presence of a bronchial carcinoma, but, of course, not of its site. Sputum, taken before breakfast, is expectorated from deep in the chest into a clean dry container. for examination by an expert cytologist. A physiotherapist can help to get a good specimen, and in those without spit inhalation of an aerosol of saline may help. Enthusiasm, attention to detail and a skilled cytologist can provide a very valuable diagnostic approach, but all three are essential for success.

## Radiology

Many patients present initially with an abnormal shadow on the chest radiograph. However, absence of radiological abnormality does not exclude bronchial carcinoma. Characteristic radiological patterns include:

1. *Collapse* (atelectasis), which is most often segmental, but frequently lobar, and can rarely include a whole lung. Collapse is usually associated with some degree of infection behind the block; this inflammatory exudate usually prevents complete collapse of the lobe, and *no* air bronchogram is seen in the collapsed lobe. The anatomical localization of the collapsed lobe is much easier when a lateral chest radiograph is available as well as a posteroanterior view (see Chapter 6).

2. *Hilar enlargement*, which may result from the tumour itself, as a central bronchial origin is common in both squamous and oat cell bronchial carcinoma, or from metastases from a more distal peripheral lesion. Enlargement of mediastinal lymph nodes, usually presenting as asymmetrical mediastinal widening, is rarely the primary radiological abnormality. Diaphragmatic palsy, with elevation of the involved diaphragm, which normally moves upwards on sniffing when screened, indicates involvement of the phrenic nerve in the mediastinum.

3. *Cavitation* of a peripheral neoplasm, which is characteristic (Fig. 70), being distinguished from tuberculous cavitation by the thick cavity wall, and the neoplastic cavity may contain a fluid level. Cavitation is most common in a squamous bronchial carcinoma. A superior sulcus tumour which appears to obliterate the apex of one lobe often also erodes an upper rib.

4. A *solitary pulmonary nodule (coin lesion)*, which may be due to bronchial carcinoma, particularly in a man over 50 year of age. Some of these patients will have symptoms such as cough or haemoptysis, and such a tumour is often over 2 cm in diameter, usually appearing in the upper lobes (see Fig. 34). It often has ill-defined markings, possibly with a spiculated pattern, but is almost *never* calcified. Other causes of such a coin lesion include tuberculoma (which may calcify) or other granulomatous conditions (Caplan's syndrome, as in rehumatoid arthritis associated with coal-worker's pneumoconiosis); a benign tumour (e.g. a hamartoma, especially if a 'popcorn' calcification is present); a bronchogenic cyst, usually appearing in men in the lower lobes; pulmonary arteriovenous fistula (lower lobes); histoplasmosis (often calcified); Wegener's granulomatosis (usually multiple); and a pulmonary haematoma (which is usually subpleural in position).

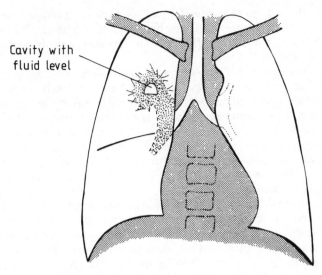

Cavity with
fluid level

*Fig. 70.*     Sketch of a posteroanterior chest radiograph with a cavitated
squamous carcinoma in the right upper lobe

Recent studies with *computerized axial tomography (CAT scan)* in
coin lesions have suggested that a relatively low radiodensity of such
lesions, as shown quantitatively by this sophisticated method, is more
likely to arise in a *coin lesion of malignant origin*, whereas higher
radiodensity (probably due to subliminal calcification) is more likely
in benign coin lesions.

In many instances the most valuable diagnostic manoeuvre in
bronchial carcinoma is to *obtain a previous chest radiograph*, and this
should always be sought. A lesion which has not changed in size over
two years is most unlikely to be malignant.

### Non-metastatic extrathoracic complications

*Neuromuscular manifestations* arise in 4–16% of cases, being commoner
with advanced disease, and usually associated with oat cell bronchial
carcinoma. Carcinomatous myopathy, myasthenia and polymyositis
are all recognized as causes of muscular weakness. A mixed peripheral
and central neuropathy is also well recognized, as is subacute
cerebellar degeneration with ataxia, incoordination and nystagmus;
rarely, dementia may occur in the absence of other neurological signs.

*Hypertrophic pulmonary osteoarthropathy* is rare, but commoner
with oat cell bronchial carcinoma. It usually presents as deep-seated
burning pain in the wrists or ankles and is associated with clubbing,

along with tenderness and swelling of the hands and wrists (and/or of feet and ankles). Subperiosteal new bone formation is seen at the ends of the long bones and can be differentiated from metastatic bone deposits by radio-isotope bone scan.

*Endocrinopathies* are usually associated with oat cell bronchial carcinoma. They seem to result from the tumour itself producing a polypeptide which either possesses hormonal activity or can release other end-organ hormones or pituitary trophic hormones. *Cushing's syndrome* (with buffalo-hump obesity, glycosuria, mild hypertension, skin atrophy with purple striae, hypokalaemia and mild poly-cythaemia) is associated with the release of ACTH activity by the tumour. This may be a 'big ACTH' which has hormonal activity although immunologically distinct from physiological ACTH. An absence of the normal diurnal variation in plasma corticosteroid levels, with a raised level which does not respond to dexamethasone suppression, is characteristic. This endocrinopathy can account for severe muscle weakness and hypokalaemic alkalosis. Treatment with metyrapone, to block the effect of the ACTH on the adrenal, can occasionally be life-saving.

The *syndrome of inappropriate secretion of antidiuretic hormone (SIADH)* presents with hyponatraemia, muscular weakness, confusion and irritability. It is usually associated with oat cell cancer and can be treated successfully with demeclocycline hydrochloride 900–1200 mg daily initially, even though the tumour itself is not responsive to treatment.

The *carcinoid syndrome* (anorexia, explosive diarrhoea and cutaneous flushing) is associated with over-production of 5-hydroxy-tryptamine, but is rare. A *hyperparathyroid* picture (to be distinguished from hypercalcaemia due to bony metastases) can give serum calcium values as high as 2.5 mmol/litre and is associated with drowsiness, polyuria and polydipsia, with marked muscle weakness. Gynaecomastia, insulin-oversecretion and calcitonin secretion have all been described in bronchial carcinoma, but are all rare.

## Diagnostic procedures

Diagnostic procedures in lung cancer are required:
 1. To establish the diagnosis.
 2. To determine the histological pattern.
 3. To determine the extent of spread of the tumour (staging).
All are necessary to plan rational treatment.

Screening procedures are applied to patients who are otherwise well and aim to determine the presence of the disease at any early stage, when hopefully curative treatment may be successful. The chest radiograph is the basis of such an approach, but recurrent chest films taken at six-monthly intervals have been shown to fail as a method of detecting cancer at a stage when treatment can affect prognosis. Large-scale and very expensive on-going trials in the USA, where sputum cytology is combined with four-monthly chest radiographs in heavy smokers aged over 45 years, is being used in an attempt to detect lung cancer at an early stage. However, the results so far suggest that the cost of finding such cases is extremely high. Positive sputum cytology, with a negative chest radiograph, then leads to extended fibreoptic bronchoscopy with the aim of localizing the tumour and thus allowing treatment.

*Bronchoscopy* (see Chapter 6) is today most commonly carried out by the fibreoptic instrument and is the major diagnostic approach in bronchial carcinoma. The bronchoscope is usually passed through the nose under local anaesthesia and allows inspection of the orifices of all 19 lobar bronchi, as well as, of course, the major bronchi, carina, vocal cords and nasopharynx. In tumours seen within the central airways, biopsy (using special forceps), brushing and suction needle aspiration are all useful in obtaining tissue for histological examination. In peripheral lesions which may beyond the vision of the bronchoscope, washings from appropriate lobar bronchi may yield positive cytological specimens. Transbronchial lung biopsy, guided by radiological screening into lesions seen on the chest radiograph, but not through the bronchoscope, may enable tissue to be obtained from these distal lesions.

*Percutaneous fine needle biopsy*, under radiological control, is now being used safely to yield tissue from more peripheral lesions. All these invasive procedures aim to produce a tissue diagnosis, so as to allow histological typing of the cancer, which is so important in planning rational therapy.

*Staging of lung cancer* relies on the Tumour, Nodes and Metastases (TNM) system, as defined by the American Joint Committee for Canger Staging. Physical examination may detect enlarged cervical or scalene nodes, liver enlargement or other distant metastases. Chest radiograph may yield evidence of local spread with barium swallow indicating mediastinal node involvement from indenting of the oesophagus, and diaphragmatic screening can show involvement of the phrenic nerve. Bone marrow aspiration can yield evidence of spread to the marrow, and the rare *leuco-erythroblastic blood film* (leucocytosis and reticulocytosis with nucleated red cells) may also indicate such spread. Aspiration of any pleural effusion with pleural biopsy can give evidence of spread to the pleura; liver scan (possibly confirmed by liver biopsy) may show evidence of tumour in that organ. Brain scanning without clinical evidence of involvement has shown to be of relatively little value.

*Mediastinoscopy and mediastinotomy*, whereby the mediastinum is explored and glands directly biopsied through a small suprasternal incision, under general anaesthesia, can yield evidence of mediastinal gland involvement and histological pattern. However, the value of this evidence of spread has been questioned, at least in attempting to decide if a squamous carcinoma is surgically resectable.

Such studies yield the following categories which can then determine the line of treatment. Small (oat) cell cancer clearly behaves differently from other types and is considered separately. Non-small cell cancer (squamous, large cell and adenocarcinoma) can be divided into:

1. *Regional disease*, which can be technically resected on surgical grounds.

2. *Limited disease*, in which surgical resection is technically impossible, but the disease is still confined to one hemithorax.

3. *Extensive disease*, with spread outwith the hemithorax.

## Treatment

### Non-small-cell cancer, regional disease

Surgical resection is possible in these patients, but unfortunately only some 20% fall into this category, but these are the only patients in whom cure is possible, although this is rare. Respiratory function in the remaining lungs or lobes, and the stage as assessed surgically at thoractomy, will determine the outcome. A preoperative $FEV_1$ below 1.5 litres, persistent hypoxaemia and/or carbon dioxide retention, cor pulmonale or severe effort dyspnoae all preclude thoracotomy. An age over 70 years, persistent pleural effusion despite repeated aspiration and involvement of the main bronchus on the left side are also usually regarded as contraindicating surgery. Preoperative radiation to a superior sulcus (Pancoast) tumour has been shown to improve the chance of surgical cure of this lesion, which is nearly always a squamous carcinoma. However, for tumours in other sites preoperative radiotherapy has proved to be of no benefit.

Chemotherapy with the drugs currently available has been shown to be of no value in squamous carcinoma and has so far only a very limited role to play in adenocarcinoma and large cell cancer. Immunotherapy, which aims to stimulate the body to reject the cancer cells as foreign cells, must still be regarded as experimental, as trials have so far been controversial.

### Non-small-cell cancer, limited disease

Surgical resection is technically impossible in these patients. The standard treatment is radiotherapy, which can produce dramatic relief of symptoms with shrinkage of tumour mass, which can allow up to 40% of such patients to survive for one year, but has a five-year survival of only 6%. Increase of the tumour dose beyond 3000 rads may yield only a little improvement in survival despite its greater power to sterilize local lesions, but this is obtained only at the cost of inducing local pulmonary fibrosis by the radiation.

## Non-small-cell cancer, extensive disease

About 50% of all lung cancer patients fall into this category, where clearly cure is impossible. The current chemotherapy regimens, using drugs either alone or in combination, have not prolonged survival of these patients. Many thus feel that symptomatic treatment alone is indicated, with radiotherapy to relieve pain from bone involvement, local cytotoxic agents (mustine, bleomycin or tetracycline) to prevent rapid recurrence of pleural effusion (see Chapter 20) and, of course, adequate pain relief by generous use of narcotics. In those patients who seem likely to survive for at least one or two months, phenol injections into the extradural space can relieve pain without the mental clouding which is produced by narcotics. This can contribute considerably to the dignity of the patient's last days.

## Small cell cancer

These tumours are both the most malignant and the most sensitive to current chemotherapy. Although most physicians feel that in this type of cancer the tumour is spread at the time of diagnosis so that surgery cannot be curative, there are occasional cases of prolonged survival following surgical resection of such tumours. Surgery should thus be considered for those isolated peripheral lesion in which no metastatic spread is shown by staging procedures. Such lesions are rarely due to oat cell cancer, the true histological nature of such lesion often being revealed only after surgicial resection.

*Chemotherapy*, using effective drugs in combination (e.g. cyclo-phosphamide, vincristine, doxorubicin, methotrexate or CCNU), has now been clearly shown by extensive controlled trials to prolong survival, particularly when used with radiotherapy to the primary lesion. However, the *possibility of cure is highly questionable* and these drugs all carry serious side effects. *Neutropenia* and rarely *thrombo-cytopenic purpura*, particularly at the early stages of treatment, can cause problems with infection and bleeding. *Haemorrhagic cystitis* is a well known complication of cyclophosphamide therapy. The patient should be warned about hair loss and wigs should be provided if needed. Vomiting and anorexia are frequent side effects of the drugs, but usually occur for only 24 hours after one pulse of combined chemotherapy (see later). These symptoms can be minimized by use of metoclopramide and cyclizine.

Prophylactic *brain irradiation* can reduce the clinical frequency of metastases to the CNS, but has not so far been shown to prolong life, as metastases at other sites still appear to remain fatal.

A *commonly used chemotherapeutic regimen* includes cyclophos-phamide (1 mg/m$^2$ intravenously), doxorubicin (40 mg/m$^2$ intravenously) and vincristine (1 mg/m² intravenously), which are given as a bolus in a well hydrated patient. The drugs are given together into a continuously running intravenous infusion which is kept up for 12 hours after the drugs have been injected. Three such pulsed courses of chemotherapy are given at three-weekly intervals, providing that the white blood count and platelet count have recovered to at least 50% of their normal values before giving the next pulse of chemotherapy.

*Doxorubicin* is cardiotoxic and should be withheld from patients with pre-existing heart disease, in whom methotrexate is substituted. The newer drug, *cisplatin* (40 mg/m²) may possibly be of value in patients with squamous cell carcinoma, but this remains to be established. The drug is given in 500 ml of half-normal saline, along with 15 mmol of potassium chloride over three hours. It is nephrotoxic and should be given only if the blood urea is below 7 mmol/litre.

It must be stressed that cure is not yet attainable by use of these drugs, but newer agents, in newer combinations, following tests by controlled clinical trials, do hold out some hope for the future. Nonetheless, present-day chemotherapy using drugs in combination can prolong life of worthwhile quality in patients with small cell lung cancer, despite one or two days of side effects every three weeks following a pulse of chemotherapy. This is particularly true in those who present with disease at a limited stage.

## Small cell cancer, *extensive disease*

The prognosis for these patients is very poor, but symptoms can demand treatment. Chemotherapy can relieve symptoms, as in superior vena caval obstruction and local bronchial obstruction, and should be considered for patients in otherwise good condition. Antibiotics (and metronidazole for anaerobic infections) can relieve the distress of 'pneumonia behind the block'. The blocking tumour itself may be at least partly removed at bronchoscopy. Other measures are similar to those used for advanced non-small-cell tumours. Sympathetic skilled nursing care is invaluable, as is the time and patience of the doctor who makes it clear that he is not abandoning his patient, merely because he cannot offer a cure.

## Conclusions

Today lung cancer is the major single problem in respiratory medicine. Obviously prevention should receive far more attention, but the promotional activities of the tobacco industry seem little hampered by the very limited effects of health education. Increased cigarette taxation, a change in the carcinogenic properties of cigarettes and intensification of efforts to prevent children taking up cigarette smoking all seem clear ways to prevent this major curse of modern man. Advances have been made in the treatment of limited disease in small cell bronchial carcinoma by chemotherapy and there is some hope of yet further advance. Nonethelesss, most cancers do not fall into this category and there is urgent need for chemotherapeutic agents which are active against squamous and adenocarcinoma. Surgery still saves a few of those afflicted with this most dreadful disease, but the overall five-year survival for all cases of lung cancer, without subdivision by histological type or stage, remains at about 5%.

# Other malignant tumours

Other malignant tumours include *bronchial adenomas*, subdivided into carcinoid tumours and cylindromata. These tumours account for less than 5% of all tumours of the lungs and most present at an earlier age than bronchial carcinoma. *Carcinoid tumours* usually present in the major bronchi, but only a small portion of the tumour is seen at bronchoscopy, most of the tumour lying outwith the bronchus. *Cylindromata* infiltrate the wall of the bronchus, often in the central airways. Cough and recurrent haemoptysis are common features of both lesions and, as with other types of bronchial neoplasm, bronchial obstruction with secondary infection is common. Both tumours are slow-growing, as are their metastases. The carcinoid syndrome is a rare consequence of bronchial carcinoid. Treatment of both tumours is primarily surgical and the prognosis is much better than that for bronchial carcinoma, particularly if any involved lymph nodes can also be removed. A *hamartoma* is a rare benign tumour, more frequent in men, usually appearing as a coin lesion with calcium distributed throughout the lesion in a 'popcorn' fashion. Local surgical excision both confirms the diagnosis and prevents the rare but recognized chance of subsequent malignant change.

### Further reading

BLEEHEN, N. (1980) The current status of management of carcinoma of the bronchus; chemotherapy and radiology. In *Advanced Medicine 16*, ed. A. J. Bellingham. Tunbridge Wells: Pitman Medical and the Royal College of Physicians of London.
GRECO, F. A. and EINHORN, L. H. (1978) *Semin. Oncol.*, **5**, 233–235
GRECO, F. A. and OLDHAM, R. K. (1979) Current concepts in cancer: small-cell lung cancer. *New Engl. J. Med.*, **301**, 355–358.
MOUNTAIN, C. F. (1977) Assessment of the role of surgery for control of lung cancer. *Ann. thorac. Surg.*, **24**, 365–373.
REULER, J. B., GIRARD, D. E. and NARDONE, D. A. (1980) The chronic pain syndrome: misconceptions and management. *Ann. intern. Med.*, **93**, 588–596.
ROYAL COLLEGE OF PHYSICIANS OF LONDON (1977) *Smoking or Health*. Tunbridge Wells: Pitman Medical.
SEYDEL, H. L. (1979) Oncology applied to diagnostic and nuclear radiology in bronchogenic carcinoma. *Appl. Radiol.*, **8**, 35–39.

STRAUSS, M. J. (1977) *Lung Cancer: Clinical Diagnosis and Treatment.* New York: Grune and Stratton.

SUDLOW, M. F. (1980) The treatment of lung cancer. In *Recent Advances in Respiratory Medicine II*, ed. D. C. Flenley. Edinburgh: Churchill Livingstone.

U.S. DEPARTMENT OF HEALTH AND HUMAN SERVICES (1980) *Health Consequences of Smoking for Women — A Report of the Surgeon General.* Washington, D.C.: U.S. Public Health Service.

YESNER, R. (1978) Spectrum of lung cancer and ectopic hormones. *Path. A.*, **13**, 217–240.

# 15

# Diffuse Pulmonary Fibrosis

A pathological increase in the fibrous tissue in the interstitial spaces of the lungs, including both the alveolar and perivascular interstitial spaces, can arise in many conditions including:

1. Pneumoconiosis, with deposition of inorganic dusts in the lungs.

2. Granulomatous disease, including sarcoidosis, tuberculosis, etc.

3. Collagen diseases affecting the lungs, as in rheumatoid arthritis, scleroderma and Sjögren's syndrome.

4. Drug-induced pulmonary fibrosis (hexamethonium nitrofurantoin, busulphan, cyclophosphamide and bleomycin).

5. Chronic pulmonary oedema, as in mitral stenosis with raised pulmonary venous pressure.

6. As late sequela of irradiation pneumonitis.

7. Lymphangitis carcinomatosis.

In all of these conditions the pulmonary fibrosis is a complication of the other disease and is usually signalled by the development of breathlessness, a rapid respiratory rate and sometimes bilateral coarse crackles at the lung bases. The chest radiograph characteristically shows diffuse bilateral reticulation, initially fine, and usually predominantly at the base of the lungs, but later progressing to coarser shadowing associated with loss of lung volume. This is shown physiologically by a restrictive pattern of respiratory function, with relatively normal $PO_2$ at rest and a low $PCO_2$, but with hypoxaemia developing on exercise.

This distinctive clinical, radiological and functional pattern of disease is usually recognized, provided that the appropriate investigations are made in the breathless patient. However, determination of the nature of the pathological process may be much more difficult. Diffuse pulmonary fibrosis is a relatively rare complication of the above diseases and in this chapter we consider two groups of conditions causing pulmonary fibrosis without any of these other primary disease processes. These are *cryptogenic fibrosing alveolitis*, and *extrinsic allergic alveolitis*. Although at present these appear to be distinct pathological processes, which can be distinguished both clinically and pathologically from the other conditions listed above, it must be realized that all such diffuse fibrosing processes tend eventually to lead to a common pathological end point known as the *end-stage lung*. It may then be impossible to determine the nature of the primary disease. At this stage the chest radiograph will show a coarse reticular or reticulonodular pattern throughout both lungs, often with cystic spaces of 3–10 mm in diameter causing the appearance of 'honeycomb lung'. When the cavities are larger than 5 mm in diameter it is likely that the process has arisen from scleroderma, histiocytosis, tuberosclerosis, rheumatoid lung or sarcoidosis.

# Cryptogenic fibrosing alveolitis

This is an uncommon disease, for the world's largest series, gathered together at the Brompton Hospital in London over many years, consists of only 220 patients. There is no strong sex preference, but the disease usually occurs in adults with a mean age around 50–60 years.

## Pathological types

Two basic pathological abnormalities are recognized; an increase in cellular thickening of the alveolar walls, which contain excess fibrous tissue, and the presence of mononuclear cells within the alveolar space.

The commonest pathological pattern of disease is known as *'usual' interstitial pneumonia (UIP)*. This is thought to start with alveolar damage causing an interstitial proteinaceous oedema, followed by monocytic and lymphocytic infiltration. Regenerated alveolar epithelial cells then cover the necrotic tissue, growing over any material that may have leaked into the alveolar space, so that such organized exudate is incorporated within the new alveolar wall. Fibrosis then develops within the alveolar interstitial spaces, often with smooth muscle proliferation. This process proceeds to the end-stage lung, with obliteration of alveoli and formation of cystic spaces lined with epithelium, giving the honeycombed appearance on the chest radiograph.

*Desquamative interstitial pneumonia (DIP)*, the less common form of fibrosing alveolitis, is characterized histologically by an accumulation of mononuclear cells in the distal air spaces. Although argument persists as to whether the same process also precedes the development of UIP, it seems that a histological appearance indicating DIP carries a more favourable prognosis than one showing UIP. As biopsies from different sites within the same patient may yield the appearances of either DIP or UIP, it is clear that the relationship between these pathological appearances and the clinical course is by no means definite. In DIP, the normal lung architecture is usually preserved, with no necrosis of alveolar lining cells; most of the mononuclear cells in the alveoli are macrophages, the remainder being proliferating desquamated alveolar Type II cells. Both UIP and DIP can progress to the end-stage lung as described above.

## Clinical features

Clinically DIP cannot be distinguished from UIP, the major features of both being progressive breathlessness, at first on effort and later at rest, sometimes with a non-productive cough and commonly associated with weight loss. Over half the patients have clubbing at presentation and this is usually an early clinical feature. On examination most patients will have bilateral basal crackles (crepitations), which occur late in inspiration, but which may vanish when the patient leans forward, indicating that the loss of lung volume is not extreme. Central cyanosis when at rest is usually a late sign and often precedes the development of cor pulmonale, which is usually a terminal event. Hypertrophic pulmonary osteoarthropathy with swelling and pain of wrists and ankles, associated with finger-clubbing, is a recognized complication.

## Radiology

Bilateral symmetrical ground-glass opacification at the lung bases is characteristic of DIP, whereas in UIP there is usually a coarser reticulonodular pattern, but in both conditions loss of volume occurs at some stage, as the disease progresses to the end-stage lung with honeycombing. However, the chest radiograph can occasionally be normal despite considerable breathlessness and a restrictive pattern in the respiratory function tests (see Chapter 1).

## Lung biopsy and bronchoalveolar lavage

Histological proof of the diagnosis can be obtained only by lung biopsy. Open biopsy at thoracotomy is justifiable only if the patient's pulmonary function is adequate and if it is thought that a histological diagnosis will decide the choice of therapy. Transbronchial lung biopsy by fibreoptic bronchoscopy is less hazardous, but carries a minor risk of inducing a pneumothorax. Multiple small biopsies can be taken, but these must be taken from one lung at a time. Alternatively, transcutaneous biopsy with a trephine drill can also yield diagnostic tissue. The new technique of bronchoalveolar lavage holds promise of increasing the understanding of the pathogenesis of these diseases, as well as giving a guide to prognosis in diffuse pulmonary disease. In this technique five or six 60 ml aliquots of buffered sterile normal saline are introduced into a basal segment at fibreoptic bronchoscopy, each aliquot then being aspirated into sterile siliconized containers. Total and differential cell counts, protein and albumin concentrations are then measured on the lavage fluid which is recovered. The procedure appears to be safe and well tolerated, occasionally producing transient pulmonary infiltrates on the chest radiograph and rarely fever and chest pain. Less than 30% of the lavage fluid is usually recovered in patients with cryptogenic fibrosing alveolitis, and in this condition fewer alveolar macrophages are obtained than those obtained by similar lavage of normal subjects. However, as in the normal subjects, alveolar macrophages from smokers are abnormal, with pigmented cytoplasmic inclusions. It seems possible that a high lymphocyte yield in the lavage fluid, to a count of over 10% of the total cells, indicates that there is a favourable outlook for treatment, whereas an increase in eosinophils or neutrophils (to over 4% of the total cells) indicates a poor prognosis, with a poor response to steroid therapy. However, these are still early results of this new investigation, which require confirmation.

## Other investigations

Clearly clinical or immunological evidence of the other conditions causing diffuse pulmonary fibrosis will be sought, for in large part the diagnosis depends upon exclusion of these other conditions. A raised ESR occurs in cryptogenic fibrosing alveolitis and a positive serum anti-nuclear factor is found in 30% of patients, whereas another 30% have a positive serum rheumatoid factor, without other evidence of rheumatoid disease. Although circulating immune complexes have been demonstrated, serum complement levels are usually normal, but IgE has been found to be deposited in the alveolar capillaries. Pulmonary function tests show a restrictive pattern, with a low transfer factor for carbon monoxide, and the shrunken lungs are stiffer than normal, even after allowing for their small volume (see Chapter 1). These patients have a tendency to develop rapid shallow breathing with hyperventilation on exercise, associated with progressive hypoxaemia as the severity of exercise increases. There is widening of the alveolar to arterial oxygen tension gradient ($A$–$aDO_2$), with a low $PCO_2$ and respiratory alkalosis at rest. Carbon dioxide retention is usually a terminal development.

## Course and prognosis

The outlook is very variable in the individual patient, so that it is very difficult to assess the value of any treatment. The mean survival can be up to three and a half years from the time of presentation, but a few patients may survive for 15 or more years. UIP usually carries a worse outlook than DIP, but variability in the histological pattern between different biopsy sites in the same patient must throw some doubt on this distinction. The radiological appearances and pulmonary function abnormalities do not correlate well with the histological pattern. Study of the type and number of cells obtained at bronchoalveolar lavage may in the future provide this missing prognostic guide. At present the individual patient may show either a rapid progression or a slow and inexorable development of disability, but rarely a relapsing and remitting pattern of disease can occur.

## Treatment

The variable prognosis makes assessment of treatment very difficult. Steroids have been used for many years and undoubtedly benefit some patients. In particular, younger patients and those who are less breathless at the time of presentation tend to respond best to steroid treatment. DIP seems more likely to respond than UIP, as an increasing prevalence of fibrosis in biopsies indicates that there will probably be a poor response to steroid therapy. Prednisolone is used in a dose of 40 mg a day by mouth, for at least six weeks in the first instance. This should be combined with potassium supplements and the usual monitoring for possible side effects (hypertension, diabetes, peptic ulceration, salt and water retention and osteoporosis). With this dosage, however, some weight gain is inevitable, but frank oedema may require diuretics. A maintenance dose of prednisolone of 10 mg/day is then reached gradually over several weeks, but recurrence of symptoms, increase of radiological opacities or further fall in carbon monoxide transfer factor and lung volumes will require further courses of higher dosage of steroids.

Although immunosuppressives are used in patients who do not respond to steroids, or in those who relapse when the steroid dosage is reduced to tolerable levels, there is no hard evidence from controlled trials that these drugs are of value and each case forms an individual therapeutic trial.

Despite much research, the cause, pathogenesis and nature of fibrosing alveolitis remain unknown. Research into collagen synthesis, protease activity and the immunological factors in lung disease may yet yield the clue to this enigma.

# Extrinsic allergic alveolitis

Extrinsic allergic alveolitis, also known as *hypersensitivity pneumonitis*, describes the lung disease resulting from a type III allergic reaction in the periphery of the lungs, centred on the alveoli, following deposition of antigenic dusts at this site. These dusts arise from animal or plant sources, including fungi and micro-organisms, and share a potential for producing allergic alveolitis if the dust particles are about 1–5 μm in diameter and can so penetrate into the alveoli. Exposure often occurs at work and the most acute responses usually follow very heavy exposure to the antigen.

The clinical pattern, course, function and radiographical abnormalities in this group of diseases tend to be very similar, irrespective of the specific antigen causing the disease.

In the United Kingdom *farmer's lung*, where the antigen is *Micropolyspora faenei* (either alone or in combination with other thermophilic micro-organisms), usually affects men of 40–50 years of age. Acute reactions tend to occur at the end of the winter, when hay which has been infected during the previous wet summer is being used for cattle feed. However, only about one-third of farm workers so exposed develop the acute reaction, but a chronic condition can lead to progressive breathlessness and cough.

In *bird-fancier's lung* the antigen is derived from avian serum proteins which are present in bird droppings and also in the dust from feathers. Pigeon fanciers are particularly at risk and their contacts may also develop the disease, even without direct contact with the birds.

Other similar conditions include *mushroom-worker's lung*, with similar antigens to those in farmer's lung; *bagassosis* where the sugar cane residue (bagasse) is contaminated by a thermoactinomycete; *humidifier pneumonitis* from contamination of water in cooling systems with pneumophilic bacteria; and *malt-worker's lung* from exposure to spores of *Aspergillus clavatus*. However, there are many other sources of similar antigens.

## Pathogenesis

The development of local symptoms of cough and dyspnoea and systemic symptoms of fever and chills, occurring some four to six hours after exposure, implies a type III immune reaction, with precipitation of antigen–antibody complexes which activate complement with consequent release of neutrophil chemotaxic factors (see Chapter 2). Specific IgE, IgA and IgM precipitating antibodies are found in the serum in most, but not all, patients and are commoner in those with the acute disease. Demonstration of such precipitins merely confirms exposure to the antigen, but does not prove that the patient is suffering from that condition. Antigen–antibody complexes are deposited in bronchiolar walls and alveolar capillaries in acute allergic alveolitis. Both immediate (five minutes to two hours) and late (four to 24 hours) immune reactions follow challenge by inhalation of the antigen. In these late reactions the lung volumes become restricted and this is often associated with fever, chills and leucocytosis, which respond to steroids, but not to beta-adrenergic drugs.

## Pathology

The *acute reaction* develops in sensitized individuals in whom antibody is already present. Antigen–antibody complexes formed with excess antigen are soluble, but still activate complement and produce local tissue damage, the infiltration of neutrophils, plasma cells and lymphocytes, along with fibrin deposition, obscuring the normal alveoli.

The *subacute stage*, some one or two months after the onset of the illness, is characterized by the development of non-caseating granulomata, similar to those seen in sarcoidosis. These are well seen in farmer's lung. 'Foam cells', consisting of histiocytes with vacuolated cytoplasm, are characteristic of bird fancier's lung. Obstructive bronchiolitis is common. The *chronic stage* develops over several months as granulomata disappear and fibrosis takes over, particularly affecting the upper lobes. Microcysts and local emphysema are frequent, leading finally to the *end-stage lung*.

## Clinical features

In the *acute form* breathlessness, dry cough and fever, associated with rigors and muscular aching, occur some two to six hours after heavy exposure to the antigen. Fine crepitations may then be widespread in both lung fields, but rhonchi are rare and there is no airways obstruction. Crepitations may persist after the fever subsides.

Continuous repeated exposure to lower concentrations of antigen, as occurs for example in budgerigar fanciers, causes gradual increasing breathlessness with associated cough and weight loss, but rarely episodic wheeze may suggest 'asthmatic bronchitis'. The weight loss can be associated with diarrhoea and jejunal villous atrophy has occasionally been demonstrated in such patients.

The disease can progress to cor pulmonale complicating the end-stage lung, as in cryptogenic fibrosing alveolitis.

## Radiology

The chest radiograph can be normal in the acute stage, but as the disease progresses, granular or nodular mottling is scattered diffusely throughout both lung fields, but mainly in the mid zones. Air space consolidation (as in pneumonia, but not showing an air bronchogram) can also occur in the acute phase, and resolves to reveal a reticulonodular pattern over a few days. Hilar gland enlargement is rare, a radiographic feature which distinguishes the condition from sarcoidosis. Repeated exposure leads to the diffuse fibrosis with loss of volume, particularly affecting the upper lobes. A honeycomb pattern is characteristic of the end-stage lung, with cor pulmonale.

## Investigations

In the acute stage arterial hypoxaemia is associated with a low $P_{CO_2}$, as in any pneumonic process, and the lung volumes may show a restrictive defect with a reduction in transfer factor. This pattern persists to the subacute stage, although in the final end-stage it may be associated with airways obstruction. In the subacute stage, where symptoms may be minimal, hypoxaemia may be revealed only by exercise, but recent further exposure to antigen can cause a restrictive pattern which resolves over two or three days following removal from the challenge.

*Serum precipitins* confirm that the patient has been sensitized to the antigen, but do not prove that the disease is present and causing his symptoms. The recently developed radio-immunoassay for antibodies can allow changes in precipitin titres to be related to antigen challenge, so giving a more precise diagnosis. Precipitins are often present in those who are exposed to the antigen, but without symptoms, and this occurs particularly in pigeon breeders, although even here precipitin titres fall slowly when these asymptomatic subjects are totally removed from the antigen.

## Management

Cure can only follow permanent removal from the antigen. Change of job is always a difficult decision and the reasons for such advice should be carefully discussed with the patient. A marked reduction in antigen exposure may be an acceptable alternative and in farmer's lung this can be achieved by such measures as drying hay before storage, substitution of silage for hay and wearing a mask fed with filtered air when in contact with the hay.

Pigeon breeders are notoriously reluctant to abandon their hobby and similar measures may therefore be needed to reduce their antigen exposure. This compromise is tolerable only in the subacute condition, for the acute condition is usually treated in hospital, so ensuring removal from the antigen. Steroids are then used initially in a dose of 40–60 mg daily, along with high concentrations of oxygen to relieve hypoxaemia. After control of the acute symptoms over one or two weeks by a high dose of steroids, these can be reduced to 10 mg of prednisolone daily for two or three months.

Farmer's lung and malt-worker's lung are prescribed occupational diseases under the British Industrial Injuries Act.

## Further reading

BERNARDO, J., HUNNINGHAKE, G. W., GADEK, J. E. et al. (1979) Acute hypersensitivity pneumonitis: serial changes in lung lymphocyte subpopulations after exposure to antigen. *Am. Rev. resp. Dis.*, **120**, 985–994.

HASLAM, P. L., TURTON, C. W. G., LUKOSKEK, A. et al. (1980) Bronchoalveolar lavage fluid cell counts in cryptogenic fibrosing alveolitis and their relation to therapy. *Thorax*, **35**, 328–339.

ROBERTS, R. C. and MOORE, V. L. (1977) Immunopathogenesis of hypersensitivity pneumonitis. *Am. Rev. resp. Dis.*, **116**, 1075–1090.

SALVAGGIO, J. E. (1979) Immunological mechanisms in pulmonary diseases. *Clin. Allergy*, **9**, 659–668.

SCHATZ, M., PATTERSON, R. and FINK, J. (1979) Immunologic lung disease. *New Engl. J. Med.*, **300**, 1310–1320.

TURNER-WARWICK, M. (1978) *Immunology of the Lung.* London: Edward Arnold.

TURNER-WARWICK, M., BURROWS, B. and JOHNSON, A. (1980) Cryptogenic fibrosing alveolitis: clinical features and their influence on survival. *Thorax*, **35**, 171–180.

# 16

# Sarcoidosis

Sarcoidosis is a systemic disorder of unknown aetiology, characterized pathologically by non-caseating epithelioid granulomata in the mediastinal and peripheral lymph nodes, lungs, skin, eyes, liver, spleen, nervous system, phalanges, parotid glands and, very rarely, heart. The epithelioid granuloma is the response of the mononuclear phagocytes to a slowly soluble antigen or irritant. In sarcoidosis the epithelioid cells forming the granuloma are in a process of rapid replacement, forming a 'high turn-over' granuloma. Demonstration of this isolated granuloma is not specific to sarcoidosis, as a similar lesion occurs in berylliosis and other conditions. However, demonstration of such granulomatous lesions in at least two distinct tissues provides a firm basis for the diagnosis of sarcoidosis.

## Epidemiology

Although half of all patients with sarcoidosis may be symptomless at the time of diagnosis, a quarter of them will have respiratory symptoms. In Britain sarcoidosis is recognized from the chest radiograph in about 10 per 100 000 cases who have a routine chest radiograph, the incidence being higher in Scandinavia and relatively low in the tropics. Symptoms (including breathlessness), signs (as of skin and eye involvement) and special investigations including hyperglobulinaemia and a positive Kveim reaction (see later) are all more prominent in black Americans than in white Americans, Britons or Scandinavians. In Britain the disease is commonest in the third and fourth decades, with a variable female predominance.

## Immunology

The tuberculin test, and other tests based on recall antigens, is depressed in sarcoidosis. This indicates a deficiency of cell-mediated T cell lymphocyte immunity, although B-cell-mediated immunity is maintained. Hypergammaglobulinaemia is also frequent. It has recently been recognized that the T cells may be reduced in the circulating blood as they are sequestered within sarcoidal lesions, at least in the lungs, from whence they can be recovered in high concentrations by bronchoalveolar lavage.

The *Kveim reaction*, which involves the intradermal injection of 0.1–0.2 ml of a saline suspension of human sarcoid tissue, following which a sarcoid granuloma develops at the site of the injection, as shown at biopsy some four to six weeks later, is widely regarded as proof of the diagnosis of sarcoidosis. A Kveim reaction is positive in about 75% of patients with acute active sarcoidosis, but the percentage of positive reaction falls as the disease becomes more chronic. In young patients with erythema nodosum and bilateral hilar adenopathy (stage I sarcoidosis, see below) the reaction is positive in some 90% of patients.

# Aetiology

The cause of sarcoidosis remains unknown. Theories of causation based on tuberculous infection, pine pollen exposure, atypical mycobacteria or fungi, and Epstein–Barr virus and involvement of genetic, occupational or social factors have all been found wanting on critical examination. The disease is commoner in monozygotic than in dizygotic twins, but there is no evidence that the HLA status is related to sarcoidosis. The recent demonstration of increased levels of *serum angiotensin converting enzyme (ACE)* in patients with active sarcoidosis is also unexplained. Nonetheless, this measurement has been used as an index of activity of the disease and thus of the need for treatment.

# Clinical features

The wide variety of tissues that can be involved in sarcoidosis indicate that the disease can present with protean manifestations, but nonetheless certain clinical patterns stand out as far more frequent than others:

1. *Bilateral hilar adenopathy* (stage I) occurs in up to 90% of patients with intrathoracic sarcoidosis. Unilateral hilar gland enlargement is uncommon, the glands usually being involved symmetrically, including the bronchopulmonary, tracheobronchial and paratracheal glands (Fig. 71).

2. *Erythema nodosum*, with painful, red purplish nodules on the front of the lower legs, is associated with bilateral hilar adenopathy in up to 50% of cases when this is due to sarcoidosis. This combination is particularly common in young women in Britain and Scandinavia, although relatively rare in North America. *Arthralgia* involving knees, ankles, wrists and elbows may also accompany erythema nodosum

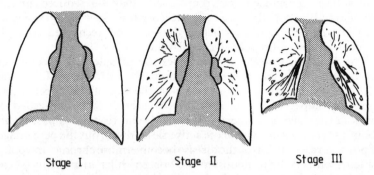

Stage I          Stage II          Stage III

*Fig. 71.*    The three stages of pulmonary sarcoidosis, as sketched from the posteroanterior chest radiograph. Stage I shows hilar adenopathy with no pulmonary involvement, stage II hilar adenopathy with pulmonary opacities, most marked in the mid and upper zones and stage III loss of volume, with marked pulmonary fibrosis, no hilar adenopathy, but one cause of the 'end stage' lung

with hilar adenopathy, as may malaise and fever. Chest pain, breathlessness and cough may also occur. Other common causes of erythema nodosum which are not associated with bilateral hilar adenopathy include primary tuberculosis, streptococcal infections and drug reactions (see Chapter 13).

3. *Lung involvement.* Radiological opacities in the lung fields may be present with hilar adenopathy, this combination being termed stage II sarcoidosis (Fig. 71). Lung involvement can develop later as adenopathy regresses. Three basic radiological patterns are recognized: the reticulonodular, the acinar and the large nodular. The reticulonodular pattern is usually a combination of a fine and coarse network, usually involving the mid zones, and only rarely associated with clubbing of the fingers or physical signs in the chest, but breathlessness and cough may be a feature. The Kveim test is positive in about 80% of such patients, but the diagnosis may also be confirmed by transbronchial lung biopsy using a fibreoptic bronchoscope. The acinar pattern, with discrete opacities of up to 6 mm in diameter, is less common than the reticulonodular pattern, but again it is usually present in the upper and mid zones of the lungs. Tuberculosis may be closely mimicked and the differential diagnosis will depend upon a positive Kveim test, a negative tuberculin test and negative sputum culture, with further proof being provided by sarcoid granulomata found on transbronchial lung biopsy. Large nodules are the rarest radiological presentation, but sarcoidosis can appear as coin lesions.

*Abnormalities in respiratory function* do not correlate well with a degree of radiological change. A restrictive pattern, with reduction in both lung volumes and TCO, is characteristic. Blood gas analysis may then show arterial hypoxaemia with a low $PCO_2$. However, this functional pattern does not distinguish sarcoidosis in any way from other lesions causing diffuse radiological opacities, which include fibrosing and allergic alveolitis and lymphatic carcinomatosis. Pneumoconiosis and metastatic cancer can also give a similar radiological picture, so that the diagnosis needs confirmation by tissue biopsy or Kveim test.

*Pulmonary fibrosis*, radiologically shown by distortion of lung tissue (Fig. 71) (stage III), with long-standing persistence of radiological abnormality, can sometimes progress to a honeycomb pattern of the *end-stage lung*. The patient then has severe effort dyspnoea, cough with eventually cor pulmonale. Emphysema, with or without reversible airways obstruction, may also complicate this terminal phase of the disease. Aspergillomata, which may cause massive haemoptysis, can develop in such emphysematous bullae or in the true cavities of the honeycomb lung. At this stage the Kveim test is positive in about a third of cases and biopsy may yield only fibrous tissue without the characteristic and diagnostic non-caseating granulomata.

## Course, prognosis and treatment

Only some 5% of patients with sarcoidosis die from the disease and this is usually from cor pulmonale, haemorrhage, aspergilloma or respiratory failure in the terminal stages of pulmonary fibrosis with the end-stage lung. Patients with myocardial sarcoidosis may present with arrhythmias and heart failure, and renal failure can result from the hypercalcaemia which is characteristic of advanced disseminated sarcoidosis. However, sarcoidosis can also cause severe prolonged disability from pulmonary or ocular involvement, without directly contributing to the patient's death.

Two-thirds of patients presenting with bilateral hilar adenopathy without lung involvement (stage I) show a complete remission of symptoms and signs within two years without treatment. Treatment with systemic steroids is thus not indicated for patients in stage I, but very florid erythema nodosum with marked systemic upset can be dramatically relieved by steroids. In patients with pulmonary involvement (stage II), which has not progressed to end-stage lung (stage III), spontaneous resolution occurs only in one-third. It is thus particularly in these patients with the stage II condition that steroids are used, although there is still no proof of their value by controlled clinical trials, so that controversy persists as to the proper role of this treatment. Protagonists of steroid therapy argue that the prevention of progression to the fibrotic stage II (end-stage lung) must improve the overall prognosis and that as steroids have been proved to resolve granulomata, they can thus prevent such progression. Similar arguments apply to the use of steroids for sarcoidosis involving other vital organs such as the eye, brain and heart.

The usual practice is thus to give steroids in a dose of 20 mg/day of prednisolone by mouth until clinical manifestations are under control, along with objective evidence of improvement. This can be shown either by radiological improvement or by serial pulmonary function tests (including the transfer factor for carbon monoxide). When such improvement is maintained, the dose can gradually be reduced to 10 mg of prednisolone by mouth daily. Initially treatment is given for six months and the steroid dosage gradually reduced thereafter if there is no rebound of activity. Some patients with chronic sarcoidosis may require life-long treatment with prednisolone.

# Non-respiratory sarcoidosis

*Eye involvement*, with uveitis, presenting as pain and mistiness of vision, presents acutely, but conjunctivitis may also be a complication of early sarcoidosis.

Erythema nodosum is the common *skin lesion*, but subcutaneous nodules and macropapular eruptions also occur. Sarcoidal lesions may develop in healed scars.

*Uveoparotid fever*, with uveitis and parotid swelling, sometimes associated with facial palsy, can be a manifestation of sarcoidosis. Symptomless *splenomegaly* is common. *Neurological lesions* include peripheral neuropathy, a space-occupying lesion in the central nervous system (including the pituitary gland) or granulomata of the cerebral vessels. The *terminal phalanges* are characteristically involved in the bony lesions, with the development of intraosseous cysts with swollen fingers. *Hypercalcaemia* is not related to the bony lesions, but hypercalcaemia is three times more common than hypercalciuria. Hypercalcaemia results from increased sensitivity to vitamin D, so that the absorption of calcium from the diet is increased. Steroid therapy rapidly corrects the hypercalcaemia, but this sometimes also occurs in hypercalcaemia arising from metastatic bone involvement by carcinoma. If hypercalcaemia is untreated, it can lead to irreversible *nephrocalcinosis* and then renal failure.

## Further reading

HUNNINGHAKE, G. W., FULMER, J. D., YOUNG, R. C. et al. (1979) Localisation of the immune response in sarcoidosis. *Am. Rev. resp. Dis.*, **120**, 49–57.

ISRAEL, H. L. (1980) Granulomatous lung disease. In *Recent Advances in Respiratory Medicine II*, ed. D. C. Flenley. Edinburgh: Churchill Livingstone.

JONES, W. W. and DAVIES, B. H. (1980) *Eighth International Conference on Sarcoidosis and Other Granulomatous Diseases.* Cardiff: Alpha Omega.

SCADDING, J. G. (1967) *Sarcoidosis.* London: Eyre and Spottiswoode.

# 17

# Occupational Lung Disease

Much of the 10 000–20 000 litres of air that an adult breathes each day is encountered at work, so that contamination of this air by dust particles (both organic and inorganic), noxious gases, fumes or vapours clearly carries the potential of causing lung disease. This will depend upon the nature of the contaminant, the degree of exposure and the susceptibility of the subject. Many of these occupational lung diseases arise insidiously and their relationship to work exposure may not be apparent at first, so that all adults with respiratory symptoms should be asked 'What jobs have you done in your working life?'.

## Definitions

*Pneumoconiosis* is defined as the accumulation of dust in the lungs and the tissue reactions to its presence. The dust is usually an aerosol of solid inanimate particles which cause either marked collagenous fibrosis (silicosis and asbestosis) or reticulin proliferation (iron, tin and barium). Organic dusts usually provoke an immune reaction, discussed under *allergic alveolitis* (see Chapter 15). Soluble gases (sulphur dioxide, ammonia, etc.) irritate the eyes and pharynx, but less soluble gases (phosgene, nitrogen dioxide, ozone, etc.) are inhaled, so causing alveolar capillary damage and pulmonary oedema. *Occupational asthma* is reversible airway narrowing caused by dusts, fumes or gases encountered at work.

## Particle deposition

Deposition of particles in the atmospheric aerosol depends mostly on size and density (see Chapter 2). Coarse mode particles (2–50 μm diameter) are mostly deposited in the nasopharynx, but fine mode (0.1–1.0 μm diameter) tend to be deposited in the alveoli. However, these small particles undergo hygroscopic growth within the airway and may impact or sediment onto the mucociliary blanket, when they may be cleared within a few hours. Particles landing in alveoli may be ingested into pulmonary alveolar macrophages or cleared by lymphatics, a process which takes days and may deposit the particles in regional lymph nodes in the hilum of the lungs.

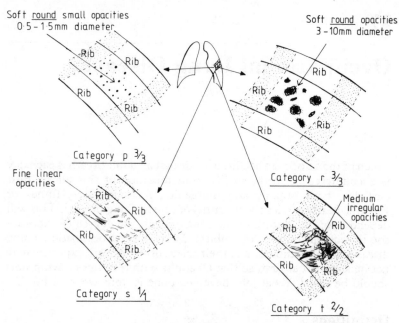

Soft <u>round</u> small opacities
0·5–1·5mm diameter

Soft <u>round</u> opacities
3–10mm diameter

Category p ⅔

Category r ⅔

Fine linear opacities

Category s ¼

Medium irregular opacities

Category t 2/2

*Fig. 72.*    Sketches of the radiographic appearances of pneumoconiosis, showing some of the categories of the ILO/UICC, as internationally agreed. The appearances are sketched from radiographs, showing the patterns in the same area of the left mid zone, just outside the cardiac outline, in four different patients

# Coal-worker's pneumoconiosis

Coal-workers pneumoconiosis is the commonest industrial disease arising from dust inhalation in Britain. Coal mining remains a very important occupation, from the number of men employed and economically, and demands for energy indicate that this will remain true for many years yet to come. Pneumonconiosis Medical Panels in Britain currently diagnose some 500 new cases of coal-worker's pneumoconiosis each year. The disease results from prolonged inhalation of coal dust particles of between 1 and 5 $\mu$m in diameter, many of which are thus deposited in alveoli and therefore ingested into pulmonary alveolar macrophages. Such overfilled pulmonary alveolar macrophages die, with release of these particles, which then join with other non-phagocytosed particles to provoke focal fibrosis locally. Dust particles are also carried in the lymphatics to the hilar lymph nodes.

In *simple coal-worker's pneumoconiosis* the chest radiograph shows many discrete opacities of 1–4 mm in size (Fig. 72), which are often

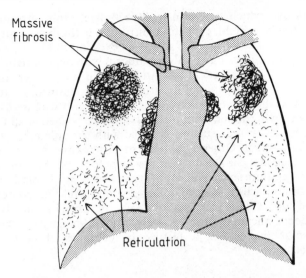

Massive fibrosis

Reticulation

*Fig. 73.*    Sketch of a posteroanterior chest radiograph in progressive massive fibrosis, showing reticulation throughout the lung fields, with dense areas of massive fibrosis, clearly demarcated from the rest of the lung fields in both upper lobes

more marked in the upper zones and may be associated with linear shadows and sometimes Kerley B lines (horizontal lines about 1 cm long lying in and above the costophrenic angles). This condition of simple coal-worker's pneumoconiosis is benign, causes no symptoms and does not impair pulmonary function or life expectancy. However, chronic bronchitis and emphysema are both very common in coal miners, but the incidence of this disease cannot be related to the presence of radiological coal-worker's pneumoconiosis. In Britain simple coal-worker's pneumoconiosis rarely arises before at least 15 years of exposure to such fine coal dust.

*Caplan's syndrome*, which can occur when rheumatoid disease coincides with simple coal-worker's pneumoconiosis, consists of development of multiple peripheral nodules, 0.5–5 cm in diameter, usually lying subpleurally and seen against a background of simple coal-worker's pneumoconiosis. On pathological section the lesions show a typical rheumatoid histological pattern and can calcify or necrose with resultant cavitation.

*Complicated pneumoconiosis* is said to occur when the simple form is associated with nodular lesions which are greater than 1 cm in diameter, often occurring peripherally and again usually in the upper lobes (Fig. 73). These lesions progress after removal of the patient from the dust, leading to the term *progressive massive fibrosis.*

Emphysema, which may also include bullae, often surrounds the nodular lesions and this probably contributes to the major symptom of breathlessness, which appears at first on exertion and later progresses to be present at rest. The $FEV_1$ is reduced, with hyperinflation of the lungs (high TLC and RV/TLC ratio), but this may be less than in a patient with similar disability from chronic bronchitis and emphysema, as the fibrotic lesions (which may be very extensive) act as a space-occupying lesion within the thorax. Hypoxaemia and carbon dioxide retention are usually associated with cor pulmonale which is often preterminal. Other symptoms in progressive massive fibrosis include haemoptysis (leading to a search for *Mycobacterium tuberculosis*, by sputum smear and culture) and *melanoptysis* (black sputum) which occurs when such a lesion cavitates and the contents are coughed up. Chest pain may be due to pleuritic involvement, spontaneous pneumothorax, or rarely from pulmonary hypertension. Finger-clubbing is *not* a feature of complicated coal-worker's pneumoconiosis.

## Management

There is no specific treatment for progressive massive fibrosis, but concomitant chronic bronchitis may be partially alleviated by bronchodilators (see Chapter 9), antibiotics for intercurrent infection, diuretics and possibly long-term oxygen therapy when cor pulmonale with hypoxaemia has become established.

In Britain *Industrial Injuries Benefit* can be claimed by a miner with pneumoconiosis. The case is reviewed by a Pneuconiosis Medical Panel, which is allowed to decide if benefit can be awarded only on the basis of the radiological appearances and the industrial history. Radiological assessment is made by the 1971 International Labour Office classification and includes:

| | |
|---|---|
| Category 1 | Small rounded opacities |
| Category 2 | Numerous small rounded opacities, but normal lung markings are still visible |
| Category 3 | Very numerous small rounded opacities, which obscure the normal lung markings |

Complicated pneumoconiosis is categorized as A, B or C, depending on the size of the opacities. Standard reference films of these categories are available for comparison (see Fig. 72). Compensation is unlikely to be paid unless at least a category 2 (simple coal-worker's pneumoconiosis) is present, as there is then a definite but small risk of the miner developing complicated pneumoconiosis.

Complicated pneumoconiosis may be prevented if miners who have developed category 2 of simple coal-worker's pneumoconiosis cease to work in an environment with such a high dust concentration. This is largely being achieved by reduction of dust concentrations in coal mines by modern industrial hygiene. Detection of category 2 pneumoconiosis by the Pneumoconiosis Medical Panel leads them to advise the miner to work in '*dust approved conditions*', where progression of disease to complicated pneumoconiosis should be prevented.

# Silicosis

Silica is widely encountered in mining of metals, quarrying, stone-dressing, casting and sand-blasting and in the pottery industry. Silica particles are strongly fibrogenic and, as with coal-worker's pneumoconiosis, this seems to depend upon silica particles being phagocytosed by alveolar macrophages, with the subsequent death of these macrophages. Pathological appearances are similar to those in complicated pneumoconiosis, but the lesions are not pigmented. Silicosis predisposes to pulmonary tuberculosis, so that progressive breathlessness, cough and episodes of 'bronchitis' in a patient working in an industry where silicosis is a recognized risk should lead to a chest radiograph. Simple silicosis shows a miliary pattern of lesions, often being more marked in the upper and mid zones of the lung fields. Complicated silicosis shows the lesions of progressive massive fibrosis, with a background of nodulation. The hilar glands, which may be enlarged, can show 'egg-shell' calcification. An acute form of silicosis can develop within six months of working in an industry with a very heavy exposure, but modern industrial hygiene should abolish such practices. There is no specific treatment for silicosis, but the patient should be removed from any further exposure to silica dust as soon as possible.

# Diseases associated with asbestos

Many people now believe asbestos to be the greatest health hazard in industry. Asbestos is a naturally occurring fibre formed by iron, magnesium, nickel and other silicates. It is resistant to fire and also to many chemicals and is therefore widely used in insulation, brake linings, electrical insulation and as an asbestos cement in buildings. There are four types of fibres: *chrysotile* (from Canada and South Africa) is the commonest; *anthophyllite*, from Italy, contains magnesium; *amosite*, from the Transvaal in South Africa, is widely used in heat insulation; and *crocidolite* (blue asbestos) is resistant to attack by acid and is mined in the Cape Province of South Africa.

The long thin fibres of asbestos tend to fall into the basal alveoli

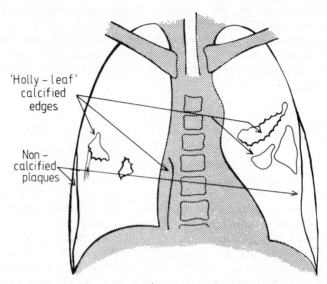

'Holly - leaf'
calcified
edges

Non -
calcified
plaques

*Fig. 74.*    Sketch of a posteroanterior chest radiograph showing multiple
bilateral pleural plaques, some partially calcified. The characteristic 'holly-leaf' pattern is seen

following inhalation, where they excite a fibrous reaction. Four
clinical syndromes are associated with exposure to asbestos.

1. *Pleural plaques* consist of collagenous deposits on the parietal
pleura, over the ribs and diaphragm. When they become calcified, they
are then easily recognized on the chest radiograph (Fig. 74). Pleural
plaques cause no symptoms and no functional impairment and
indicate merely that the patient has been exposed to asbestos. Rarely
pleural effusions can be associated with residual fibrosis of the visceral
pleura and then the development of a restrictive defect of respiratory
function. Uncalcified pleural plaques are the commonest radiographic
manifestation of asbestos exposure, calcification usually developing
only some 20 years after the patient was first exposed to asbestos.

2. *Asbestosis* is legally defined as pulmonary fibrosis due to inhalation of asbestos. Breathlessness is the dominant symptom. Finger-
clubbing is common and is associated with bilateral coarse basal
crepitations or crackles. The radiographic signs are most prominent in
the basal regions and start with a ground glass appearance, but develop
into a reticular pattern of linear opacities obscuring the heart and
diaphragmatic borders, eventually extending to involve most of the
lung fields (Fig. 75). Pleural plaques may coexist and there may
occasionally be homogeneous opacities which are greater than 1 cm in

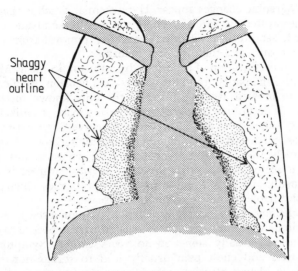

*Fig. 75.*   Sketch of a posteroanterior chest radiograph in asbestosis, showing diffuse pulmonary fibrosis, with the characteristic 'shaggy' outline to the heart border

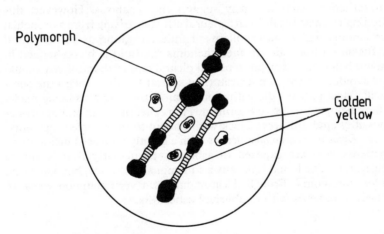

*Fig. 76.*   Sketch of asbestos bodies as seen in the sputum

diameter. *Asbestos bodies* (Fig. 76), which consist of an asbestos fibre surrounded by a coat of golden-brown pigment, with bulbous ends, may be recognized in the sputum, but indicate only that the patient has been exposed to asbestos and have no other diagnostic value. A restrictive pattern of pulmonary function is characteristic, the carbon monoxide transfer factor (TCO) usually being reduced, even before overt radiographic changes appear. Hypoxaemia, which is character-istically aggravated by exercise, develops as the disease advances. Once established, asbestosis progresses even after removal from further asbestos exposure and the disease is incurable.

In Britain certification of asbestosis by a Pneumoconiosis Medical Panel entitles the patient (and his widow) to a pension. Reduction in exposure to inhaled asbestos fibres is the only known method of prevention. The unique properties of asbestos make it unlikely that industry will abolish its use. However, alternative fibres with similar physical properties which are made of glass, molten rock or slag are being actively investigated as substitutes for asbestos, but unfor-tunately, it seems possible that the very physical properties which make the material desirable may also be those properties which render the particles liable to induce respiratory disease.

3. *Mesothelioma* is an incurable malignant tumour of the pleurae (or rarely peritoneum), most strongly associated with exposure to croci-dolite asbestos, usually some 20–40 years earlier. Symptoms of breathlessness and chest pain usually lead to recognition of the characteristic pleural effusion, which may obscure the underlying neoplasm. Alternatively, nodular opacities on the periphery of the lung and the mediastinum appear. The mediastinum is not shifted to the contralateral side by the pleural effusion associated with a mesothelioma and this may suggest the diagnosis. However, this finding can also result from a pleural effusion arising from a bronchial carcinoma, which causes collapse of underlying lung, as well as pleural effusion on that side. In mesothelioma the fluid is blood-stained in about half of all cases, but repeated pleural taps or thoracotomy should be avoided, as the tumour can then spread locally through the chest wall. Most patients die within one year of the diagnosis being made, there being no curative treatment. Pain relief may demand opiates or possibly epidural nerve block with phenol to the affected segments.

4. *Bronchial carcinoma* occurs with a greatly increased incidence in patients who are exposed to asbestos, particularly if they smoke cigarettes. The lesion is usually a squamous carcinoma, but may be an adenocarcinoma. Bronchial carcinoma is a very common cause of death in patients with established asbestosis.

# Occupational asthma

Asthma caused by materials encountered at work is now being recognized more frequently. Avoidance of the causative agent may prevent further attacks, both in the presenting patient and in future in his work-mates. Any patient with asthma should therefore be asked about his work.

*Recognized causes* include colophony, which is the flux in soft solder used in the electronics industry; wood dust, particularly western red cedar; grain mites, in farmers and workers in the food industry; *Bacillus subtilis* enzymes, in biological washing powder manufacturing; drugs, including penicillin and methyldopa in the pharmaceutical industry; chemicals, such as di-isocyanates, as in the plastic foams manufactured for the furniture industry; some paints and lamination adhesives; epoxy resins in adhesives; and the complex salts of platinum in refining of this metal.

Symptoms include wheeze, cough and breathlessness which can be related to work within a few minutes or hours of exposure to the causal agent. The symptoms characteristically improve at weekends or holidays, although in delayed reactions, such as those due to iso-cyanates, the symptoms may not resolve within a single weekend.

The $FEV_1$ may be normal between attacks, as when the patient is seen at an out-patient clinic, as for example in other types of asthma. If a careful history leads to suspicion of an occupational cause, this can usually be proved only by recording the peak expiratory flow when at work. Measurements of PEF should ideally be made every two hours for two weeks when at work, followed by two weeks away from work, without using any drugs during this period to control the asthma. If this ideal is unattainable in practice, normal recordings over two weeks, including a weekend away from work, would tend to make the diagnosis of occupational asthma extremely unlikely. Bronchial challenge to the suspected agent causing the asthma may also be necessary to confirm the diagnosis and, as this can carry important implications for an industry, such a test may be justifiable if the patient agrees. The usual precautions should be taken, of course, with careful medical supervision and availability of hydrocortisone and bronchodilators. Observation for at least 12 to 24 hours should be made, as a delayed reaction to the potential causal agent may occur.

Identification of a patient with occupational asthma can imply that other workers, exposed to the same industrial environment, are also at risk. This is particularly important where the agent has not previously been identified as causing occupational asthma and clearly the continual introduction of new materials into industrial processes makes this very likely to continue to occur in the future. However, even old industries such as farming can yield new discoveries. Thus, grain mite asthma has been defined only within the last few years. Unfortunately, skin prick tests and identification of circulating precipitins are still at the research stage and are not yet reliable enough for use in clinical diagnosis. Thus, the only certain method to establish a diagnosis of occupational asthma is the tedious prolonged recording of peak flow measurements, as described above. The worker must be loaned a peak flow meter and shown how to use it for this to be carried out satisfactorily.

*Treatment* preferably means removal from exposure to the causal agent. Drug treatment with bronchodilators, including inhaled sympathomimetics, oral steroids and disodium cromoglycate is often inadequate if heavy exposure continues to occur at work. A compromise, whereby drugs to prevent asthma are associated with a reduction in exposure, without necessarily abolishing all exposure, may be acceptable to an individual patient, if change of his job is impracticable.

## Further reading

KANNERSTEIN, M., CHURG, J. and ELLIOT McCAUGHEY, W. T. (1978) Asbestos and mesothelioma: a review. *Path. A.*, **13**, 81–129.
MORGAN, W. K. C. and SEATON, A. (1975) *Occupational Lung Diseases.* Philadelphia: W. B. Saunders.
MUIR, D. C. F. (1980) Occupational lung disease. In *Recent Advances in Respiratory Medicine II*, ed. D. C. Flenley. Edinburgh: Churchill Livingstone.
NEWMAN TAYLOR, A. J. (1980) Occupational asthma. *Thorax*, **35**, 241–245.

# 18

# Diseases of the Pulmonary Circulation

## Structure and function of the pulmonary circulation

The pulmonary circulation allows the total cardiac output of 5–8 litres/minute in the resting adult to perfuse most of the 300 million alevoli in the normal lungs with a pulmonary arterial pressure of only 20/8 mmHg, giving a total pulmonary vascular resistance of less than 200 dyne.cm.sec$^{-5}$. The right ventricle, which lies under most of the praecordium on clinical examination, only the apex beat being formed by the left ventricle, has a much thinner wall than that of the left ventricle, for this latter must maintain the systemic arterial pressure, some six times higher.

The *pulmonary arterial trunk* and main pulmonary arterial branches are elastic vessels, but branches with a diameter of less than 0.5 cm are muscularized, although like all pulmonary arteries they are thin-walled. The pulmonary arterioles, with a diameter smaller than 70 $\mu$m, have no muscle and only a single elastic lamina. The networks of alveolar capillaries occupy most of the alveolar walls, with an average diameter of about 8 $\mu$m, pulmonary blood flow usually perfusing several alveoli before entering the pulmonary venules. Larger venules, which lie within the interacinar fibrous septa, are thin-walled and have an irregular elastic lamina. The pulmonary veins contain no valves.

The *bronchial arteries* are systemic vessels arising from the aorta, which after entering the lung form an anastamoses around the hilum, thereafter giving branches which supply the bronchi as far as the respiratory bronchioles and thus also provide a supply to most types of lung neoplasms, including bronchial carcinoma. Bronchial arteries also supply hilar lymphatics and branches of the vagus nerve within the lungs. Anastamoses between the bronchial and pulmonary arteries are common in infancy, but become less frequent in the adult. However, there are numerous communications between the pulmonary and bronchial *veins*, within the bronchial venous plexuses.

The *lung lymphatics* are very extensive, starting as blind sacs at the respiratory bronchioles and reaching towards the hilum through interacinar fibrous septa. They play an important role in health in preventing pulmonary oedema by absorbing excess fluid from the alveolar interstitial spaces (see Chapter 22).

# Pulmonary thromboembolism

Embolization of the pulmonary arterial tree by a thrombus is found in up to 20% of routine hospital autopsies. The thrombus usually arises from the deep veins of the legs and is most often undetected clinically in life. Virchow's triad — venous stasis, local injury to the intima of the vein and an ill-defined hypercoagulable state — remains as the recognized mechanism leading to such venous thrombosis. All these conditions arise postoperatively, in pregnancy, particularly post-partum, or in patients lying in bed, particularly those with congestive heart failure. Burns and fractures to the lower limbs are other well recognized factors, as are increasing age, obesity, contraceptive pills containing a high dose of oestrogens and the immobility of a leg resulting from a hemiplegia. The clot, which starts in the sinuses behind the venous valve, can become detached and float in the blood stream, through the right heart, to lodge in a pulmonary artery or its branches. The consequences then depend upon the size of the vessel occluded, the patient's previous cardiopulmonary status and the activity of the fibrinolytic system which proceeds to dissolve the clot.

*Venous thrombosis* occurs particularly in the deep veins of the calf, where it *may* cause calf tenderness, ankle oedema and a positive Homan's sign (pain in the calf on dorsiflexing the ankle). However, few or none of these signs are present in most cases. Iliofemoral thrombosis carries a greater risk of pulmonary embolism, but again may be silent. Alternatively, local tenderness over the groin or anteroposterior aspect of the thigh, with swelling and increase in skin temperature of the affected leg, may give a clue, particularly if associated with distension of superficial veins.

Intravenous injection of $I^{131}$-labelled fibrinogen leads to deposition of label within the newly formed clot, so that a localized accumulation of radio-activity can be detected by external scanning of the legs. However, the diagnosis can only be proved by *venous angiography*, which shows a clear filling defect if a clot is present in the veins. These methods have shown that 50% of venous thromboses are clinically silent and develop *during or immediately after surgery*, and not several days postoperatively as formerly thought. Most importantly, such thromboses can be prevented by low-dosage heparin both before and after surgery. Heparin is injected subcutaneously in a dose of 5000 units two hours preoperatively; this dose is repeated eight- or 12-hourly for five to ten days or until the patient is fully ambulant. Contraindications to such therapy include aspirin, even if taken for five days preoperatively, and, of course, oral anticoagulants!

The *physiological consequences of pulmonary embolism* include reflex tachycardia, hyperventilation, arterial hypoxaemia and a low arterial $P_{CO_2}$. Continued ventilation of the poorly perfused alveoli which are distal to the embolic occlusion causes further local hypocapnia, which appears to induce local bronchoconstriction, thus reducing the ventilation to the embolized area. The hypoxaemia correlates reasonably well with the extent of an embolic occlusion. Hypoxaemia may result from shunting through a patent foramen ovale, if there is severe pulmonary hypertension, or from a fall in cardiac output or increase in perfusion to poorly ventilated alveoli. Local pulmonary atelectasis is a late result, arising from local loss of surfactant which serves to maintain alveoli distended. Lysis of the clot by the plasminogen–plasmin system probably requires release of plasmin activator from the intima of the occluded pulmonary vessel, with lysis occurring over four to 14 days, but then there is further slow clearing of the clot up to six weeks after the initial embolic event.

*Pulmonary infarction* is an uncommon consequence of pulmonary embolism, as the bronchial circulation and the patent airway still provides oxygenation of the lung tissue which lies distal to the site of embolism.

*Clinical features* depend on the size of embolus and on the time of the event. Massive pulmonary embolism with occlusion of the main pulomonary arterial trunk is a classic, but rare cause of sudden postoperative death. The sudden onset of severe breathlessness with tachycardia, hypotension and central cyanosis, possibly associated with wheeze and a gallop rhythm on auscultation of the heart, may be found in those cases with less dramatic pulmonary occlusion. The most usual symptom is breathlessness of sudden onset. Pleuritic chest pain and haemoptysis are *relatively uncommon* symptoms and probably indicate pulmonary infarction which may be associated with a blood-stained pleural effusion. Tachycardia is usual. Arrhythmias, such as atrial fibrillation, ectopic beats or transient heart block, can occur and a major occlusion can produce a right ventricular lift and a loudly split second heart sound in the pulmonary area, but this sign tends to disappear when the cardiac output falls in massive occlusion. In most patients occlusion is less severe and such signs are often absent.

The *plain chest radiograph* is usually normal in the acute phase and rarely shows ischaemia of an affected lung zone. The major value of the radiograph at this stage is to exclude other possibilities such as pneumonia as the cause of the symptom. Pulmonary infarction may be associated with a raised diaphragm on the affected side and a small pleural effusion. A linear shadow, usually in the lower zones, indicates the 'plate atelectasis' developing later in the course of pulmonary thromboembolism (Fig. 77). The ECG usually shows a tachycardia and 'non-specific T wave changes'. P pulmonale, right axis deviation

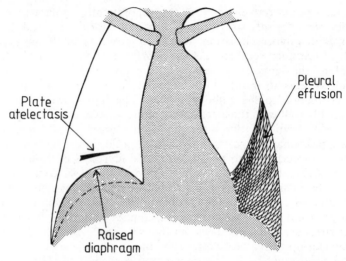

*Fig. 77.*    Sketch summarizing the possible radiographic appearances in pulmonary infarction; these include a raised diaphragm on the affected side, atelectasis, and/or a pleural effusion (here shown on the opposite side for clarity)

and an $S_1Q_3$ configuration and inverted T waves in the anterior chest leads are characteristic, but by no means invariable (Fig. 78). The alveolar to arterial oxygen tension gradient ($A-aDO_2$) is usually widened, as the arterial $PCO_2$ is low even if the arterial $PO_2$ appears to be normal on first inspection.

The *perfusion scan*, in which the distribution of a gamma emitter ($I^{131}$ or $Tc^{99m}$ technetium), which is tagged onto intravenously injected microspheres and imaged within the lung fields by a gamma camera, is the most useful specific investigation, short of pulmonary angiography. The microspheres injected intravenously are about 35 $\mu$m in diameter, but they lodge in the pulmonary arterioles or even capillaries for the latter are only some 8 $\mu$m in diameter. However, they will lodge only in those areas where the blood flow carries them to the site of lodgement, so that filling defects in the lungs on lung perfusion scan appear in the areas of pulmonary embolism where no blood flow is occurring. It must be emphasized that similar appearances can arise in *many other lung conditions*, notably pneumonia, but there the filling defect on the perfusion scan coincides with an opacity on the plain chest radiograph. In emphysematous bullae, or in bronchial asthma, filling defects will appear on the perfusion scan, without corresponding opacities on the chest radiograph. In asthma such appearances can resolve rapidly within a few hours, but caution should always be used in interpreting perfusion scan appearances in a patient who is known to

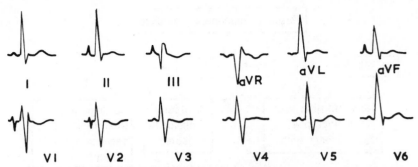

*Fig. 78.* ECG appearances in pulmonary embolism. Note tall peak P waves, partial right bundle branch block (rSr in $V_1$), S in lead 1, QS and negative T in III and inverted T waves in $V_1$–$V_3$. (*From D. G. Julian (1978) Cardiology. London: Baillière Tindall*)

have a low $FEV_1$. The perfusion lung scan therefore has most value diagnostically in a patient who had a normal chest radiograph and a normal $FEV_1$ at the time of the scan. A normal perfusion scan then effectively rules out significant thromboembolic obstruction.

A *ventilation scan*, using a radio-active gas, usually xenon 133 (or preferably krypton 81m if available), may also show that ventilation is reduced to the regions of poor perfusion. However, the poor resolution (particularly with radio-active xenon), combined with the physiological mechanisms which reduce the ventilation to alveoli whose blood supply is obstructed, mean that such ventilation/perfusion scans rarely add much diagnostic precision. Parenchymal lung disease (pneumonia, bullous emphysema, diffuse fibrosis), whilst reducing perfusion, often also reduces ventilation to the same areas of the lungs.

*Pulmonary angiography* provides the most specific diagnosis of thromboembolism. Despite initial hesitancy, the technique is now known to be safe even in patients with severe obstruction of the pulmonary circulation, provided that resuscitation equipment is available. Radio-opaque dye is injected through a cardiac catheter into the main pulmonary artery at first, and this is then usually followed by selective angiography, particularly directed to those areas of the lungs where a filling defect is identified on the perfusion scan. Measurements of the pulmonary vascular pressures and the cardiac output can be made before the angiogram, through the same catheter in the pulmonary artery, so as to define the haemodynamic consequences of the embolization.

By using pulmonary angiography as the definitive proof of pulmonary thromboembolism in life, it has now become apparent that the disease is, in fact, less common than previously suspected on the basis of post mortem evidence. It seems probable that pulmonary embolism

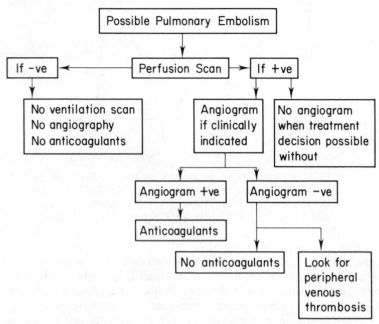

*Fig. 79.*    Decision tree for the treatment of pulmonary embolism

can arise as part of the process of dying from any prolonged disease process, and such patients will usually be immobile, in heart failure with other known precipitants of venous thrombosis. It now seems probable that the pulmonary circulation, even in health, is continually being obstructed on a microscopical scale by repeated small emboli, which are promptly lysed. Clinical pulmonary thromboembolism thus only results when such lysis fails, presumably often because the clot is too large.

Diagnosis of pulmonary thromboembolism will usually lead to treatment with anticoagulants which does carry some hazard of bleeding, and this risk is considerably greater if thrombolytic therapy is used, where cerebral haemorrhage has been recorded. Diagnosis also carries implications for contraceptive advice and life insurance, and a possible threat of recurrence, but clearly a decision in diagnosis is much to be desired. Unfortunately, this can be very difficult. A management decision tree for patients suspected of having pulmonary embolism on clinical grounds is shown in Fig. 79, illustrating the logical sequence of steps which are recommended.

## Management

The management of pulmonary embolism depends upon the severity and rapidity of onset of the disease.

*Massive pulmonary thromboembolism* will usually present as cardiac arrest and suspicion that this has arisen from pulmonary thromboembolism may arise from an obvious deep venous thrombosis or in a patient with a known risk factor. External cardiac massage, combined with mouth to mouth breathing are the emergency measures, followed as quickly as possible by cuffed endotracheal intubation and ventilation with high concentrations of oxygen, with continuation of the cardiac massage. Intravenous bicarbonate therapy should be cautious, as obviously the venous circulation can rapidly be overloaded if the pulmonary circulation is occluded. Rarely these measures can sustain life for long enough to allow a *surgical embolectomy* to be undertaken, using cardiopulmonary bypass, but most surgeons will require a diagnostic pulmonary angiogram before undertaking this heroic procedure.

*Less dramatic embolization* requires oxygen in high concentrations, intravenous heparin in a dose of 10 000–15 000 units intravenously, initially, continued with a slower constant intravenous infusion of 20 000–30 000 units over 24 hours. Alternatively, four doses of 5000–10 000 units can be given intravenously for 24 hours. Digoxin may be necessary for atrial arrhythmias. Fibrinolytic therapy using streptokinase through an indwelling pulmonary arterial catheter is theoretically attractive, but has considerable problems in practice as the material is antigenic. The human fibrinolytic agent urokinase does not have this draw-back, but is extremely expensive and in a controlled trial in the United States was found to have no significant advantage in outcome over treatment with heparin alone.

After initial heparinization, anticoagulation is continued with oral warfarin, usually starting some four or five days after the initial event, as the heparin dosage is tailed off. Warfarin is started in a dose of 15–30 mg on the first day (depending on body weight), 10–20 mg orally on the second day, the dosage thereafter being controlled to ensure that the prothrombin time lies between two and three times the control value. The duration of warfarin therapy has not been clearly established by controlled trials, but most physicians would continue this treatment for at least six weeks after a definite embolic event, but for longer if the factor initiating the original venous thrombosis continues. Contraindications to prolonged warfarin therapy include a proved bleeding peptic ulcer, liver disease with endogenously impaired prothrombin synthesis or an unreliable patient. Untoward bleeding in a patient maintained on warfarin can be controlled by stopping the warfarin or reversing its effects with vitamin K1 (10–15 mg). It is important to recall that warfarin may be displaced from its binding to plasma proteins by diuretics, oral antidiabetic agents and anti-inflammatory agents; dosage must therefore be adjusted in the light of prothrombin time if these other drugs are also given. Warfarin is metabolized in the liver by microsomal enzymes, these enzymes being induced by drugs such as barbiturates and phenathiazines, again requiring an adjustment of warfarin dosage to maintain a satisfactory prothrombin level.

Prevention of recurrence of further pulmonary thromboembolism from the legs by the partial occlusion of the vena cava (using a Michel clip or plication) is controversial and is little used today, as complications, including venous ulceration of the legs and persistent oedema, are by no means infrequent.

# Thromboembolic pulmonary hypertension

Although most pulmonary emboli are successfully lysed by the body's plasmin–plasminogen system, occasionally recurrent small emboli appear to exhaust the lung's capacity for lysis and the emboli become organized and permanently occlude the pulmonary circulation. These patients often present without clear recognition of previous episodes of pulmonary embolism or infarction, but complain of exertional breathlessness, which may be associated with anginal pain and occasional episodes of syncope on effort. Right ventricular hypertrophy is indicated by a parasternal heave, with a loud pulmonary second sound, and an enlarged heart on chest radiograph. These signs may precede the development of overt congestive heart failure, with elevated jugular venous pressure and peripheral oedema. Right ventricular hypertrophy may be confirmed by ECG and pulmonary arterial catheterization confirms pulmonary hypertension, often with an impaired response of the cardiac output to exercise. Hypoxaemia and a low $P\text{CO}_2$ in the arterial blood are characteristic, but lung volumes and $FEV_1$ are usually normal. Ventilation/perfusion scan may show multiple filling defects and pulmonary angiography can confirm the diagnosis. Prolonged anticoagulation with warfarin is indicated, along with digoxin and diuretics as necessary to control heart failure. The major differential diagnosis is from primary pulmonary hypertension.

# Other pulmonary emboli

Other pulmonary emboli include *fat embolism*, characteristically seen 12–36 hours after bony injury, with breathlessness, tachycardia, delirium and fever, sometimes associated with multiple petechiae over the thorax and upper extremities. Chest radiography shows bilateral widespread small opacities, as in other types of adult respiratory distress syndrome (see Chapter 11). Patients show central cyanosis and arterial blood analysis confirms hypoxaemia with a low $P\text{CO}_2$, at least initially. Fat may be present in the sputum and urine. The treatment is as for other causes of the adult respiratory distress syndrome. *Amniotic fluid embolism* should be suspected in a woman who develops sudden dyspnoea, central cyanosis and hypotension following spontaneous or caesarean delivery. *Tumour embolism* may closely mimic pulmonary thromboembolism, but the symptoms and signs fail to remit despite anticoagulation. *Foreign bodies* introduced into the venous circulation can also embolize to the lungs and these include plastic intravenous tubing or the irritant agents used to dilute heroin which is injected intravenously by 'main-lining' drug addicts. Ova and cysts of *Schistosoma* may embolize to the lung where they can cause granulomatous reactions around the vessels, with the resultant vasculitis producing serious pulmonary hypertension.

# Primary pulmonary hypertension

This is a disease of unknown aetiology characterized by right ventricular hypertrophy, without other heart abnormality, raised pulmonary artery pressure being associated with a normal pulmonary wedge pressure. There are no other known causes of pulmonary hypertension present. The disease occurs most commonly in young adult females. The appetite suppressant, aminorex, which is not available in the UK, caused a minor epidemic of this disease in 1967–70 in German-speaking Europe. Dyspnoea on exertion is invariable in patients with primary pulmonary hypertension, with anginal pain on exercise and effort syncope also being characteristic symptoms. Central cyanosis, with peripheral cyanosis and cold extremities from the low cardiac output, is associated with the parasternal heave of right ventricular hypertrophy. A loud pulmonary second sound suggests pulmonary hypertension and this can be confirmed by cardiac catheterization, where mean pulmonary arterial pressures of 40–80 mmHg are usual, with marked right ventricular hypertrophy being shown on ECG. Pulmonary vasodilatation has only been attained in this condition by use of intravenous isoprenaline, but this is of little use for continuous treatment of this otherwise fatal condition.

## Further reading

BIELLO, D. R., MATTAR, A. G., McKNIGHT, R. C. and SIEGEL, B. A. (1979) Ventilation–perfusion studies in suspected pulmonary embolism. *Am. J. Roentgenol.*, **133**, 1033–1037.

MOSER, K. M. (1979) *Lung Biology in Health and Disease, 14. Pulmonary Vascular Diseases.* New York and Basel: Marcel Dekker.

ROBIN, E. D. (1977) Overdiagnosis and overtreatment of pulmonary embolism: The Emperor may have no clothes. *Ann. intern. Med.*, **87**, 775–781.

SABISTON, D. C. (1979) Pathophysiology, diagnosis and management of pulmonary embolism. *Am. J. Surg.*, **138**, 384–391.

# 19

# Collagen Vascular Disease and the Lungs

Collagen vascular diseases are disorders of unknown aetiology, which are usually chronic and characteristically involve more than one organ system in the body. The diseases themselves are relatively rare, or the pulmonary involvement in the common diseases (e.g. rheumatoid arthritis) is uncommon, but they do carry importance as in many instances pulmonary involvement may come to be the major threat to life, and in some of these conditions specific therapy can now greatly improve the prognosis.

## Wegener's granulomatosis

Wegener's granulomatosis is an uncommon disease of later adult life, with granolomatous angiitis involving the upper respiratory tract (nose and paranasal sinuses), lung and kidneys. Arthralgia and persistent purulent nasal discharge with crusting may be the main symptoms, associated with cough and sometimes haemoptysis. The chest radiograph shows single or multiple round opacities, which can cavitate and characteristically come and go as the disease progresses. Microscopic haematuria and proteinuria indicate renal involvement. Proof of the diagnosis depends upon adequate biopsy, which is not always obtained from nasal lesions. Immunological involvement is shown by the high ESR, fever and circulating immune complexes. A dramatic response can be obtained to a combination of oral prednisolone with an immunosuppressant drug such as cyclophosphamide or azathioprine. These drugs may need to be continued for months or years and, as such therapy carries definite risks, as with any immunosuppression, this is only justifiable if the diagnosis of Wegener's granulomatosis is firmly established by pathological examination of an adequate biopsy specimen.

## Polyarteritis nodosa

Polyarteritis nodosa is a rare disorder in which a patchy necrotizing vasculitis involving all the coats of small muscular arteries can occur in the arteries in any organ, but the kidneys are involved in over 80% of cases. The lungs (usually the bronchial arteries) are usually only involved in about 30% of cases. The pathological lesions contain immunoglobulin and complement, but the exact immunopathology has not been established. Infection with hepatitis B virus (HBV) or streptococci and drugs (penicillin, sulphonamides, etc.) have all been implicated in the causation of polyarteritis nodosa, but it also seems that some host factor is operating in addition. Polyarteritis nodosa can present clinically with asthma (which may be chronic) and is associated with blood eosinophilia and episodes of pneumonia with cough and haemoptysis. Weight loss and hypertension are common features, the frequent renal involvement being shown by microscopic haematuria and proteinuria. A rheumatoid type of arthropathy is characteristic and neurological involvement classically presents with mononeuritis multiplex. Appearances on the chest radiograph are very variable. There may be no abnormality, but patchy pneumonic infiltrates which are bilaterally asymmetrical and tend to wax and wane are probably the most characteristic appearances on the chest radiograph.

Biopsy of an affected vessel, or renal biopsy, can prove the diagnosis. Treatment with corticosteroids combined with azathioprine may prevent the otherwise relentless progression, often with death occurring within a few months of presentation in untreated cases.

# Rheumatoid disease

Rheumatoid disease can involve far more than merely the joints, as shown by the following manifestations in the respiratory system.

*Pleurisy*, with or without effusion, is the commonest respiratory lesion in rheumatoid disease, the effusions often being associated with subcutaneous nodules and high titres of rheumatoid factor in the serum (and pleural fluid). The effusions are characteristically chronic and may be bilateral. The glucose concentration in the pleural fluid is usually lower than that in simultaneously drawn venous blood. A high cholesterol concentration is usual in such effusions, as in those with any chronic condition, and this gives the pleural fluid a shimmering appearance. Fluid usually recurs after aspiration and there is a recognized risk of producing a chronic bronchopleural fistula if the lung is damaged by attempts at pleural aspiration in these patients.

*Necrobiotic nodules* appear on the chest radiograph as masses which can be up to 7 cm in diameter, multiple or solitary, and usually based close to the pleura. They are characteristically asymptomatic, but can cavitate. Cough and haemoptysis can then be associated, as can pleural effusion and subcutaneous nodules. Lung nodules tend to wax and wane over the years.

*Caplan's syndrome* is the name given to multiple round opacities of diameter 0.5–5 cm, seen in the periphery of the lungs, with a background of category 0 or 1 simple *coal-worker's pneumoconiosis*, along with the joint involvement of rheumatoid arthritis. The lesions can cavitate and have a characteristic histological appearance with a central necrotic zone, surrounded by pallisaded fibroblasts. The presence of coal dust in the nodules is characteristic of the Caplan lesion, but this is not found in the necrobiotic nodules of rheumatoid disease. Rheumatoid factor is always strongly positive in patients presenting with Caplan's syndrome.

*Diffuse interstitial pulmonary fibrosis* is a rare but recognized complication of rheumatoid disease, usually being associated with clubbing of the fingers and basal crackles. Subcutaneous nodules are also common in such patients, but the clinical features are otherwise similar to those in patients presenting with diffuse pulmonary fibrosis, but without rheumatoid disease (see Chapter 15).

# Systemic lupus erythematosus

Systemic lupus erythematosus (SLE) is a multi-system disease associated with circulating immune complexes. Inflammatory changes develop in blood vessels of connective tissue and on serous surfaces throughout the body; the kidney is often involved. The lungs and pleura are involved in about 50–70% of patients, particularly when the disease is extensive. Painful pleurisy with effusion is common, often occurring during an exacerbation of the condition. Pleural effusions may be recurrent and are often bilateral, the effusion being an exudate. However, unlike rheumatoid effusions, the pleural fluid glucose is not lower than that of simultaneously drawn venous blood (see Chapter 20). Bilateral basal atelectasis is common, and may be associated with involvement of the diaphragm by systemic lupus erythematosus. Lupus pneumonia is associated with fever, tachypnoea and hypoxia, with patchy bilateral alveolar infiltrates on the chest radiograph. Diffuse interstitial lung disease, although recognized in systemic lupus erythematosus, is less common than in rheumatoid disease. Breathlessness when lying down may indicate involvement of the diaphragm, which is associated with a reduction in lung volumes, due to an inability to take a full inspiration.

# Sjögren's syndrome

Sjögren's syndrome is a chronic inflammatory disease in which the patient usually presents with a dry mouth, dry eyes and drying of other mucous membranes, along with a rheumatoid type of arthropathy. As in rheumatoid disease, pleurisy, with or without effusion, is common, but the most serious complication is recurrent persistent pneumonia. This results from drying up of the tracheobronchial secretions, so that inspissated mucus causes atelectasis with subsequent infection. Steroids may sometimes relieve this bronchiolar obstruction.

# Ankylosing spondylitis

Ankylosing spondylitis is a chronic inflammatory disease, principally affecting the central joints of the body, and is almost confined to men. A rheumatoid type of peripheral arthropathy occurs in up to one-third of cases. The disease classically presents with back pain in a young man, and the radiograph shows a sacro-iliitis. An HLA B27 histocompatibility phenotype is found in 90% of Caucasian patients with ankylosing spondylitis. Anterior uveitis and aortic insufficiency are recognized complications. Pulmonary involvement includes chest wall restriction from *fusion of costovertebral joints* and upper lobe *fibrobullous disease*. The lung volumes are minimally restricted, but the FRC is often increased, with relative preservation of the $FEV_1$, as the chest fixes at a high lung volume. Fibrobullous disease probably occurs in less than 10% of patients with ankylosing spondylosis, but starts as apical pleural thickening and progresses to apical interstitial infiltrate, which then breaks down to form a cavity. Both upper lobes can be involved, so that tuberculosis can be closely mimicked. The cavities can become infected with *Aspergillus*, forming a mycetoma (see Chapter 22), and this may precipitate massive haemoptysis. Fibrobullous disease often progresses slowly, usually only complicating long-standing ankylosing spondylosis. Patients with pulmonary involvement from ankylosing spondylosis are at risk if they require a laparotomy for an incidental surgical condition, for they depend largely upon the abdominal muscles in the diaphragm to provide spontaneous ventilation.

# Goodpasture's syndrome

Goodpasture's syndrome, in which antibody-mediated rapidly progressive glomerulonephritis is associated with haemoptysis and diffuse pulmonary infiltrates due to the alveolar haemorrhage, results from a circulating antibody to glomerular basement membrane. This anti-GBM cross-reacts with the alveolar basement membranes. IgG antibody is deposited along both glomerular and alveolar membranes and can also be found in the circulation. Treatment with prednisolone (60 mg/day) and immunosuppressants (cyclophoshamide 3 mg/kg/day and azathioprine 1 mg/kg/day), along with daily plasma exchange to remove circulating antibody, has been successful in treatment, particularly in controlling pulmonary haemorrhage. Repeated plasma exchange can lower the circulating antibody to undetectable levels, when the antibody does then not subsequently reappear.

# Idiopathic pulmonary haemosiderosis

Idiopathic pulmonary haemosiderosis presents as recurrent haemoptysis (often causing iron-deficiency anaemia), with cough and breathlessness in children and young adults. A fine nodular infiltrate is present on the chest radiograph, resulting from blood and haemosiderin filling some alveoli. Some patients survive for many years, but others die within three or four years of the first symptom. The rheumatoid factor in the serum can be positive and some cases have a deficiency of IgA, but the immune basis for the disease has not been established. Correction of the iron-deficiency anaemia can improve the breathlessness, but pulmonary fibrosis, which is presumed to result from the haemosiderin deposits, appears to be little influenced by steroids or immunosuppressives.

## Further reading

HUNNINGHAKE, G. W. and FAUCI, A. S. (1979) Pulmonary involvement in the collagen vascular diseases. *Am. Rev. Resp. Dis.*, **119**, 471–503.
ROSENBLATT, S. G., KNIGHT, W., BANNAYAN, G. A. et al. (1979) Treatment of Goodpasture's syndrome with plasmapheresis. *Am. J. Med.*, **66**, 689–696.
SALVAGGIO, J. E. (1979) Immunological mechanisms in pulmonary diseases. *Clin. Allergy*, **9**, 659–668.
YEAGER, H., POWELL, D., WEINBURG, R. M. et al. (1976) Idiopathic pulmonary haemosiderosis. *Archs intern. Med.*, **136**, 1145–1149.

# 20

# Diseases of the Pleura

## Pleural effusion

### Physiology of the pleural fluid

In health, fluid continually moves across the pleural space, driven by the systemic capillary hydrostatic pressure, aided by the negative intrapleural pressure, both opposed by the oncotic pressure of plasma proteins which remain in the capillary, after subtracting the oncotic pressure of the pleural fluid proteins (Fig. 80). These forces thus favour the formation of a pleural fluid. However, the pulmonary capillaries have a lower hydrostatic pressure ($10 \, cmH_2O$), so favouring absorption of the fluid through the visceral pleura. These forces depend upon the healthy capillary endothelium preventing the passage of large plasma protein molecules, so that any fluid formed in response to such forces is a *transudate* (or *hydrothorax*), which usually has a protein concentration of less than 30 g/litre. Such a transudate will increase in volume if there is a rise in the systemic capillary hydrostatic pressure (congestive heart failure) or pulmonary venous pressure (pulmonary oedema) or if there is a fall in plasma oncotic pressure (hypoproteinaemia from cirrhosis, nephrotic syndrome, etc.). Rarely, a hydrothorax can be associated with ascites in a benign ovarian tumour (Meigs' syndrome) and a hydrothorax is also a rare complication of myxoedema, when the fluid clears only with thyroxine therapy.

However, if an inflammatory process damages the capillary endothelial cells, with disruption of their intercellular connections, so allowing large molecules to pass from the capillaries, the fluid-retaining property of the plasma proteins no longer operates across this semipermeable capillary membrane. Fluid can then rapidly accumulate in the pleural space. In this circumstance, however, the fluid is an *exudate*, with a protein concentration of over 30 g/litre. Similar circumstances apply if there is obstruction to the lymphatic drainage of the pleura, which can again cause accumulation of a pleural fluid with high protein concentration.

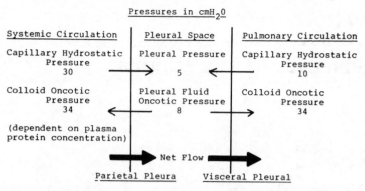

*Fig. 80.* Pressures driving the fluids across the pleural space

## Differentiation of transudates from exudates

Differation of these two types of effusion on the grounds of the protein concentration alone will lead to error in classification of about 10% of cases, but if the lactic dehydrogenase (LDH) levels in the fluid are also measured, this inaccuracy is reduced. On this basis *transudates have*:

1. A ratio of the pleural fluid protein concentration to plasma protein concentration of more than 0.5.

2. A ratio of the pleural fluid LDH level to the serum LDH level of more than 0.6.

3. A pleural fluid LDH level which is more than two-thirds of the upper limit of the normal LDH serum level.

## Clinical features

Breathlessness may be the only symptom resulting from pleural effusion, but pleuritic pain, haemoptysis and cough may be caused by the underlying condition leading to the effusion, as may fever and toxaemia, particularly when the effusion is an exudate.

The classical physical signs of an effusion are diminished movement on the affected side, stony dullness to percussion (which may be higher in the axilla than over the front or back of the chest) and absent breath sounds over the fluid. Aegophony (a nasal bleating quality to the spoken sound as heard through the stethoscope) may be present at the upper level of the fluid. Effusion of at least 500 ml is necessary to produce these signs, but a very large effusion may also displace the apex beat and rarely the trachea to the opposite side.

The *chest radiograph* classically shows a diffuse opacity, which is most dense at the pleural surface and higher laterally (see Fig. 33). This appearance arises from the cylindrical nature of the chest and does not necessarily mean that more fluid is present in the lateral aspect. The costophrenic angles are obscured even by a small effusion and if this is not loculated it is usually seen on the lateral radiograph to lie in the posterior vertebrophrenic angle. Loculated effusions may occur anywhere within the thorax, but are much commoner towards the bases. They may also accumulate in the lung fissures, with radiographic thickening of the fissures. A chest radiograph taken in the lateral decubitus position shows that a non-loculated pleural effusion lies in the most dependent zone of the lungs, thus along the lower lateral chest wall, and this radiograph can be particularly helpful in distinguishing a pleural effusion which lies over the diaphragm. Such an effusion is otherwise very difficult to distinguish from an opacity caused by a raised hemidiaphragm.

*Ultrasound* can distinguish a pleural effusion (where the echos from the parietal and visceral pleura move apart asymmetrically with respiration) from an encysted fluid lying within the lung parenchyma, as in lung abscess, for in this condition the echos from the inner and outer edges of the mass together move symmetrically with respiration.

Absolute proof of the presence of a pleural effusion depends upon *thoracentesis*. This is carried out over the site of maximal dullness to percussion, usually with the patient seated and the aspiration carried out over the back of the chest. After skin preparation, and infiltration of local anaesthetic, an initial exploration is made with a fine needle which has injected the local anaesthetic, thus obtaining fluid. This diagnostic tap is then followed by aspiration through a wider gauged needle, particularly if the fluid is very turbid, as in an empyema. No more than 1 litre of fluid should be removed initially and less if this is adequate to relieve breathlessness. Pulmonary oedema can occur in a re-expanded lung, for reasons which are not well understood. Failure to obtain fluid at thoracentesis often results from attempting the aspiration through an intercostal space which is too low.

A *pleural biopsy* with Abrams' punch is a valuable diagnostic aid, but this must be carried out before the fluid is aspirated. The punch is inserted through a small stab wound in the chest wall, following local anaesthesia (Fig. 81). After the punch is in the pleural space a little fluid is aspirated and the punch is then angled so that the notch lies on the side of the parietal pleura. The whole punch is then gradually withdrawn until the notch is felt to catch on the parietal pleura; the punch is then briskly closed, so obtaining a specimen of parietal pleura. The whole punch is then withdrawn in the closed position. Three or four biopsies from different angulations of the punch at the same site can be taken safely and these increase the yield of diagnostic tissue.

Complications of pleural biopsy include production of a pneumothorax and some minor bleeding. Biopsy should not be carried out if the patient is known to have a bleeding tendency, unless this is first corrected. The cause of an effusion can be determined in up to 60% of

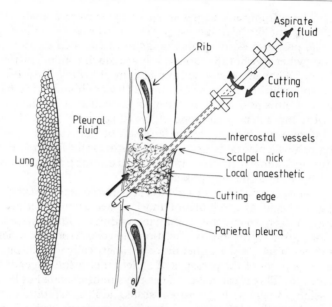

*Fig. 81.*   Pleural biopsy using Abrams' punch. The punch can be angled
laterally, both before and backwards, so as to obtain several
different bites and pleural biopsy specimens through the same
insertion in the chest wall. However, the cutting edge of the punch
must always be directed inferiorly, towards the upper end of the
rib below the insertion, so as to avoid the intercostal vessels

cases from the results of biopsy, but this can rise to up to 80% in cases
of tuberculous pleural effusion.

## Causes

The commonest causes of pleural exudates are:

1. *Post-pneumonic pleural effusion*, classically following bacterial
pneumonia, but rare with viral pneumonia. An amber- or straw-
coloured fluid is obtained, which is slightly cloudy and on microscopy
is seen to contain a large number of polymorphonuclear leucocytes.
The fluid is usually sterile, as the pneumonia will usually have been
treated with an appropriate antibiotic previously. A low pH ($<7.20$) in
a post-pneumonic pleural effusion is an indication that an intercostal
tube drainage is likely to be needed, as the effusion proceeds to form an
empyema, with very turbid fluid which cannot be adequately aspirated
through a needle.

2. *Post-pneumonic empyema*, although rare today, is a recognized
complication of pneumonia, notably that due to *Staphylococcus
pyogenes* or *Strep. pneumoniae*. Empyema is classically associated with

recrudescence of fever, pleuritic chest pain following the initial pneumonia, and the patient is clearly toxic with weight loss. Aspiration yields frank pus, which may be thin in an acute empyema, but later becomes thick as the empyema becomes chronic and may be thus very difficult to drain through such a needle, so that intercostal tube drainage is then required.

3. A *malignant pleural effusion* usually arises from bronchial carcinoma, directly seeding into the pleural space; secondary spread from breast cancer or Hodgkin's lymphoma is also possible. Rarer malignant causes of pleural effusion include metastatic tumour from other sites, e.g. pancreas, stomach and ovary, or *pleural mesothelioma* associated with exposure to asbestos (see Chapter 17). Malignant effusions are characteristically blood-stained and tend to recur after initial aspiration. The protein concentration is high and the glucose low in about 15% of cases. Malignant cells are identified in about 60% of malignant effusions, but their differentiation from the normal pleural mesothelial cells requires an expert cytologist. Malignancy can also cause pleural effusion to occur by obstruction of lymphatics, without necessarily direct tumour invasion of the pleural space. As little as 1 ml of blood can render 500 ml of a pleural effusion apparently blood-tinged, with pleural fluid red cell counts then being between 5000 and 100 000/mm$^3$. Blood originating from a traumatic tap will not cause any macrophages in the pleural fluid to contain haemoglobin inclusion bodies and recognition of these bodies, which stain pink with Wright's stain, thus implies that there is a pathological cause for the presence of the blood in the fluid.

4. *Pulmonary infarction* may only declare on the chest radiograph as a pleural effusion, this characteristically being of small volume and blood-stained; the diaphragm is often raised on the affected side. Eosinophils may constitute up to 50% of the cell content of the effusion. However, such eosinophilia of pleural fluid is often associated with a blood-stained effusion of any origin and is not diagnostic of pulmonary infarction.

5. *Tuberculous pleural effusion* results from tubercular protein gaining access to the pleural space of a sensitized patient. Primary tuberculous pleural effusion is now rare, but classically had a peak incidence in adolescence and was rare in patients under five years of age, but usually occurred within one year of the primary tuberculous infection. Pleuritic pain, with an acute onset associated with fever and malaise, is the characteristic feature of a tuberculous effusion, and the tuberculin test is strongly positive. The pleural exudate contains lymphocytes as the predominant cell type. Culture of large volumes of the pleural fluid, after concentration, may yield *Mycobacterium tuberculosis*, but the diagnosis may be more rapidly established by identification of pathological tubercles in the pleural biopsy specimen.

The tuberculous pleural effusion of adolescence may heal with fibrosis, with resultant impairment of respiratory function. If untreated, about one-third of such patients will develop pulmonary tuberculosis within five years of the pleural effusion.

In post-primary pulmonary tuberculosis intrapleural rupture of a tuberculous cavity can produce a *tuberculous pyopneumothorax* and a tuberculous empyema can arise from intrapleural rupture of a paravertebral cold abscess.

6. *Rheumatoid arthritis* can cause pleural effusion, which is often bilateral and persistent over many years, being particularly common in men with rheumatoid disease. As with any chronic effusion, the cholesterol concentration is high, giving a characteristic shimmering appearance to the aspirated fluid. Rheumatoid factor is usually present in the serum (and in the pleural fluid) and subcutaneous nodules may be present. Rheumatoid pleural effusion is asymptomatic in about one-third of cases. The protein concentration and lactate dehydrogenase level in the fluid are both high, but the glucose concentration is characteristically lower than that in a simultaneously taken venous blood sample. However, this reduction in glucose concentration in the fluid also occurs in about 15% of malignant effusions and also in post-pneumonic effusions which are actively infected. The presence of immune complexes in the pleural effusion is a newly described feature, very suggestive of the presence of active rheumatoid disease. The pH of such rheumatoid effusions is often below 7.20.

7. In other *collagen vascular disorders*, e.g. systemic lupus erythematosus (SLE), polyarteritis nodosa, Sjögren's syndrome, etc., pleural effusions are recognized complications, these occurring most commonly in SLE (see Chapter 19). The pleural effusions of systemic lupus erythematosus are characteristically bilateral, often associated with pleuritic pain, and may occur at any stage of the disease, but most often during an exacerbation of the lupus. Although a post-pneumonic pleural effusion can be mimicked clinically, the glucose concentration in the fluid is not lower than that of the plasma in systemic lupus erythematosus and LE cells are sometimes found in the pleural fluid.

8. *Pancreatitis* can cause a pleural effusion which is usually left-sided. Such an effusion will have a very high amylase concentration, usually very much higher than that in simultaneously taken venous blood. Rupture of the oesophagus, or pleural malignancy, can also raise the serum amylase level in the pleural fluid.

## Treatment

*Hydrothorax* (a pleural effusion which is a transudate) usually responds to diuretics, but thoracentesis may be needed to relieve urgent breathlessness. Oxygen administration is desirable for such patients as the pleural effusion further impairs gas exchange, so aggravating the hypoxaemia, which is usually combined with a low $P_{CO_2}$, as a characteristic feature of patients with congestive heart failure. In hypoproteinaemia, hypoxaemia can also arise from shunting of blood through unventilated alveoli behind the closed airways at the bases of the lungs.

Treatment of a *pleural exudate* depends on the cause. Postpneumonic effusions are usually sterile and may require only one thoracentesis, the pneumonia being treated with antibiotics. Empyemata may be aspirated to dryness when the fluid is thin and appropriate antibiotics may be continued until the fluid has completely resolved. Aspiration may be repeated two days later, but when the fluid becomes viscid it is difficult to aspirate through the needle and under-water sealed drainage through an indwelling intercostal tube is required. Chronic empyemata, which are rarely seen if antibiotic therapy of a pneumonia has been adequate, may require thoractomy and decortication of the underlying lung, with resection of the empyema space and of the surrounding thickened pleura, so allowing the lung to expand.

Cure of *malignant pleural effusions* is clearly impossible. Distressing breathlessness, which recurs as the fluid reaccumulates after the initial thoracentesis, demands relief. A host of agents have been used over the years to try and prevent such re-accumulation of fluid. At present tetracycline (500 mg diluted in 30–50 ml saline), given through a chest drainage tube, appears to be the most effective and to have the fewest side effects. The older regimen of nitrogen mustard (20 mg diluted in 40 ml saline), injected into the pleural effusion, after an almost complete aspiration at thoracentesis, is effective, but associated with nausea and vomiting. Chest pain, fever and leucopenia are also recognized complications of nitrogen mustard. Immunotherapy with *Corynebacterium parvum* instilled into the pleural fluid has recently been suggested as an effective means of preventing reaccumulation of malignant effusions, with very few side effects. Pleural effusions arising in Hodgkin's disease usually respond well to local radiotherapy.

*Tuberculous pleural effusion* requires antituberculous chemotherapy as discussed in Chapter 13. This should be associated with prednisolone (40 mg/day initially, then dosage declining over six weeks), given by mouth, to prevent residual pleural fibrosis.

# Empyema thoracis

An empyema thoracis means pus in the pleural cavity. This most commonly results from pre-existing lung infection, usually a bacterial pneumonia (including tuberculosis), but lung abscess and bronchiectasis are also recognized causes. More rarely, empyema arises from chest wounds, or as a complication of thoracic surgery, or oesophageal rupture (where the empyema is left-sided). Much more rare causes include rupture of a subphrenic abscess, osteomyelitis of a rib, as a part of a septicaemia, actinomycosis, or from rupture from a hepatic amoebic abscess.

*Pathologically*, deposition of fibrin on the pleural surfaces from the purulent effusion eventually results in a thick-walled abscess containing pus. At the earliest stage the fluid is cloudy, but frank pus suggests that the fluid is becoming encysted. An untreated chronic empyema progresses to a frozen chest with unilateral elevation of the diaphragm and local rib fixation as the fibrous capsule of the encysted empyema slowly contracts. The underlying lung is poorly ventilated, so contributing little to gas exchange.

*Clinically*, the development of an acute empyema is usually suggested by the reappearance of a low-grade fever several days after apparent successful treatment of a bacterial pneumonia, combined with signs of a pleural effusion. Aspiration of pus from the pleural space confirms the diagnosis. Organisms are often not cultured in the fluid if the primary infective process (pneumonia or lung abscess, etc.) has been treated with antibiotics, but pneumococcal antigen may be present in the fluid, indicating its origin in a *Strep. pneumoniae* infection. Anerobic organisms may be found if appropriate culture methods are used. The pus should also be cultured for *M. tuberculosis*, unless there is definite evidence that the underlying lung infection was not tuberculous.

*Radiologically*, a non-encysted empyema appears as any other pleural effusion. An encysted empyema has a characteristic D or oval shape, based on a lung boundary, often with a clearly defined border (Fig. 82). On both posteroanterior and lateral films a mediastinal tumour (ganglioneuroma, see Chapter 23) may be mimicked.

A *bronchopleural fistula*, where the empyema space communicates with the bronchial tree, can cause large quantities of pus and blood to be coughed up, with a pyopneumothorax being shown by a fluid level in the pleural space.

*Management* depends upon providing adequate drainage, combined with high doses of appropriate antibiotics. Needle aspiration, which may be repeated every second day, may be adequate if the fluid remains cloudy, but when the needle yields frank pus, an intercostal drain is required. If the pus is thick and viscid, a resection of a portion of rib is necessary to ensure adequate drainage. Chronic empyema, which usually results from delay in diagnosis or mismanagement of the acute stage, is best treated by decortication, with complete excision of the empyema space and its surrounding fibrous tissue, so freeing the underlying lung. Alternatively, in a patient not fit for such major surgery, prolonged drainage over several months may eventually be successful. If a postoperative empyema complicates resection for

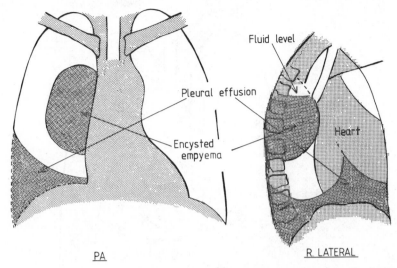

*Fig. 82.*   Sketch of posteroanterior and lateral chest radiographs in a patient with an encapsulated empyema of the right pleura. A right pleural effusion (non-encapsulated) is also present

bronchial carcinoma, the prognosis may be improved, possibly as some ill-understood stimulus causes immunological mechanisms to reject tumour metastases elsewhere in the body. Gas seen radiologically in previously opaque hemithorax following pneumonectomy always suggests that a bronchopleural fistula has developed.

# Pneumothorax

*Spontaneous pneumothorax* occurs most commonly in men, being some six times more common than in women; most patients are aged between 15 and 40 years of age. Another peak incidence occurs in patients with chronic bronchitis and emphysema, usually who are over 50 years of age. As most cases resolve spontaneously, the exact cause is usually undetermined. However, rupture of a pleural bleb at the apex of the lung is usually blamed and recently such single blebs have been shown by scanning electron microscopy to show a deficiency of normal pleural mesothelial cells. However, it is not yet clear if this appearance results from presence of air in the pleural space or is itself the primary cause of the leakage of air. Classically, young patients with spontaneous pneumothorax have no associated disease and their lungs are otherwise normal. However, spontaneous pneumothorax can complicate lung disease. This occurs in asthma (where an undetected tension pneumothorax can be fatal); pulmonary infarction; bronchial

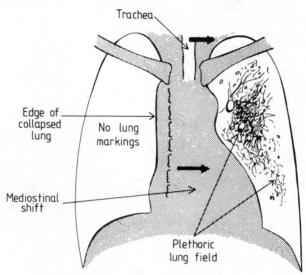

*Fig. 83.*   Sketch of the posteroanterior radiograph in a patient with a right tension pneumothorax, causing marked mediastinal shift, as indicated by position of the trachea, and the heart, the vertebral bodies forming the edge of the mediastinal shadow from apex to base. The opacity lying next to the vertebral shadows in the right side is the collapsed right lung, and there is increased plethora in the left lung field, where all the cardiac output goes. No lung markings are apparent in the translucent right hemithorax

carcinoma (where the air leak may persist despite under-water sealed drainage); pneumonia (particularly staphylococcal); cystic fibrosis; and diffuse pulmonary fibrosis of whatever aetiology (see Chapter 15).

*Traumatic pneumothorax* is a well recognized complication of rib fracture, but the fracture may not always be evident on the initial chest radiograph. Iatrogenic traumatic pneumothorax from malposition of a central venous catheter is a well recognized hazard. Alveolar rupture causing pneumothorax is a known hazard of artificial ventilation with positive end-expiratory pressure (PEEP). Respiratory collapse during induction of anaesthesia should always raise the suspicion of a pneumothorax, which may be under tension.

## Clinical features

Spontaneous pneumothorax presents as a classical picture in a young man, who is suddenly taken with a severe, unilateral chest pain, associated with breathlessness which may become progressively worse. On examination the most important physical sign is absence of the breath sounds, usually over one apex. The percussion note may be

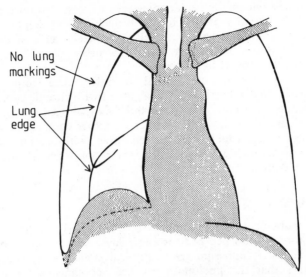

No lung markings

Lung edge

*Fig. 84.* Sketch of the posteroanterior radiograph of a right pneumo-thorax, showing the lung edge, with partial collapse of under-lying lung and no mediastinal shift. The fissures between the lung lobes are clearly seen

normal, possibly hyper-resonant, and very rarely can be impaired. It is therefore an unreliable sign of pneumothorax. The dangerous *tension pneumothorax* can lead to systemic hypotension with progressive hypoxia and a falling cardiac output. This results from impairment in both venous return to the right side of the heart and in pulmonary gas exchange. A tension pneumothorax is recognized from the history of progressive breathlessness and should therefore be suspected before the signs of shift of the apex beat and/or trachea away from the side of the pneumothorax develop.

The *chest radiograph* confirms the diagnosis of pneumothorax (Fig. 83), even a minor degree of which produces a clear area without lung markings, contiguous to the ribs (Fig. 84). The lung edge is often clearly apparent on close inspection of the film under a bright light. The underlying lung is thus collapsed to a greater or lesser degree, but only becomes radio-opaque when the collapse is almost complete. A posteroanterior radiograph taken in *full expiration* in the erect position may reveal a pneumothorax which is not otherwise apparent on the normal film taken in full inspiration.

Hypoxaemia is rarely significant in the spontaneous pneumothorax of young adults, when ventilation/perfusion ratios tend to be pre-served, as the partially collapsed lung has a similar reduction in blood flow. However, a large pneumothorax can cause hypoxaemia with a low $P_{CO_2}$ and widened alveolar to arterial oxygen tension gradient (A–a$DO_2$). In a patient with chronic bronchitis and emphysema a spontaneous pneumothorax is a well recognized cause of type II respiratory failure (see Chapter 11), when carbon dioxide retention complicates the arterial hypoxaemia.

A pneumothorax may be difficult to differentiate from a *large emphysematous bulla*, particularly in a patient with chronic bronchitis and emphysema. A clear rim to the bulla may be seen on the chest radiograph and thus allow the distinction. Other common causes of acute chest pain, which may be confused with a spontaneous pneumothorax, include myocardial infarction, pneumonia and pulmonary embolism.

## Treatment

A small spontaneous pneumothorax in a previously healthy young adult requires merely bed rest for a few days, until breathlessness is relieved and it is apparent from physical signs and radiographic appearances that the pneumothorax has spontaneously resolved. However, when more than 20–30% of the pleural space on one side is occupied by air, under-water sealed drainage is recommended. This is established by insertion of an intercostal drain, usually in the fourth or fifth intercostal space, behind the anterior axillary line, under local anaesthesia. If adhesions are present at this site, an alternative is the second intercostal space in the anterior chest wall. The tube is removed some 24–48 hours after the under-water sealed drain has ceased to bubble. The drainage bottle must never be raised above the patient, otherwise the water in the seal will drain into the pleural space! A second drain may be required if bubbling persists. If the deflated lung still cannot be re-expanded, a thoracic surgical opinion should be sought as operative intervention may be necessary.

A chest drain is painful and analgesia should be adequate whilst the drain is in place; opiate narcotics can be used if there is no danger of carbon dioxide retention.

The emergency treatment of a tension pneumothorax is by insertion of a needle of as wide a bore as immediately available through the chest wall. A hiss of escaping air proves the diagnosis and can relieve a life-threatening emergency. However, it is preferable, if possible, to attach the needle to a smoothly moving all-glass syringe, which is held half-filled with air. If the plunger moves in as the needle enters the pleural space, intrapleural pressure is clearly negative, whereas if the plunger moves outwards, a tension pneumothorax is proved. More formal intercostal drainage with an under-water sealed drain can follow relief of the severe emergency.

Recurrence of a spontaneous pneumothorax on the same side suggests that there is a persistent anatomical defect. Most physicians would agree that such a recurrence on the same side on three separate occasions is an indication for considering *pleurectomy*, whereby the parietal pleura is stripped surgically from the chest wall. This is very effective in preventing recurrence of a pneumothorax and respiratory function is usually unimpaired following such a procedure. However, pleurodesis may also be secured by pleural abrasion at a limited thoractomy or by insertion of *iodized talc* (or kaolin) into the pleural space through an intercostal drain, the aim of both methods being to ensure irritation of the pleural surfaces, without infection, yet sufficient to maintain adhesion of the parietal and visceral pleura.

*Complications* of a pneumothorax include severe bleeding into the pleural space, which may require an emergency thoractomy. Infection, with development of a pyopneumothorax, requires aspiration and antibiotics and possibly later surgical resection if a chronic empyema results. Purulent sputum is also an indication for antibiotics in a patient with a spontaneous pneumothorax.

# Further reading

AUSTIN, E. H. and FLYE, M. W. (1979) The treatment of recurrent malignant pleural effusion. *Ann. thorac. Surg.*, **28**, 190–203.

HALLA, J. T., SCHROHENLOHER, R. E. and VOLANAKIS, J. E. (1980) Immune complexes and other laboratory features of pleural effusions. A comparison of rheumatoid arthritis, systemic lupus erythematosus and other diseases. *Ann. intern. Med.*, **92**, 748–752.

HIRSCH, A., RUFFIE, P., NEBUT, M., BIGNON, J. and CHRETIEN, J. (1979) Pleural effusion: laboratory tests in 300 cases. *Thorax*, **34**, 106–112.

LIGHT, R. W. (1977) Pleural effusions. *Med. Clins N. Am.*, **61**, 1139–1352.

LOWELL, J. R. (1977) *Pleural Effusions: A Comprehensive Treatise*. Baltimore: University Park Press.

# 21

# Adverse Effects of Drugs on the Lungs

Respiratory disease can result from side effects of drugs which have often been given for non-respiratory disorders. Common examples of such disorders are the following.

## Bronchoconstriction

Beta-adrenoreceptor blocking drugs ($\beta$-blockers) include acebutolol, atenolol, metoprolol, nadolol, oxprenolol, pindolol, propranolol, sotalol, and timolol. All these drugs can cause a small but definite fall in $FEV_1$, even in normal subjects, but this effect can be much greater in patients with asthma or chronic bronchitis and emphysema. Beta-blockers are commonly prescribed for the treatment of angina or hypertension and the underlying asthmatic tendency may be either ignored or disclosed only when breathlessness becomes apparent. Airways obstruction is confirmed by a low $FEV_1$, low $FEV_1/FVC$ ratio and low peak expiratory flow; it usually returns rapidly to normal when the beta-blockers are withdrawn. All beta-blockers appear to have this effect in some degree, but it is possible that the *cardioselective drugs* (acebutolol, atenolol and metroprolol) may be less likely to produce this bronchoconstriction than the non-selective beta-adrenergic receptor blocking drugs propranolol, oxprenolol, timolol, sotalol and pindolol.

In practice it is best to avoid the use of any beta-blocker in a patient with airways obstruction, but if there is a strong indication for the drug, such as a cardiac arrhythmia or severe and otherwise intractable angina, one of the cardioselective agents should be used cautiously, with monitoring of the $FEV_1$. Increase in airways resistance from beta-blockers can usually be reversed by a $beta_2$ stimulant such as salbutamol or terbutaline. This may need to be given in relatively large doses and, of course, tends to reverse the other $beta_2$ effects of the beta-blocker. Patients known to have airways obstruction or hypersensitive bronchi probably have their hypertension treated with methyl dopa, with or without a diuretic, and it is possible that nifedipine 10 mg three times daily by mouth may be the best choice for treatment of angina in patients with airways obstruction.

*Histamine release*, inducing asthma, can rarely result from *analgesics*, including morphine and pentazocine, or from muscle relaxants including tubocurarine, suxamethonium and pancuronium. Any general anaesthetic given to an asthmatic or chronic bronchitic patient should thus take account of these potential interactions. *Aspirin* and the related tartarzine (a yellow coloured dye) can induce asthma by inhibition of prostaglandin synthesis (see Chapter 10).

# Diffuse pulmonary infiltrates

*Methotrexate* is a widely used antimetabolite for treatment of acute lymphoblastic leukaemia, as well as tumours of breast, head and neck and osteosarcoma. It is also used in the treatment of psoriasis. Methotrexate can cause diffuse bilateral interstitial pulmonary infiltrates, which are clinically associated with breathlessness, cyanosis and cough, occurring 12 to 200 days after starting the treatment. Blood eosinophilia is common, implying a hypersensitivity reaction. Hypoxaemia with a low $P\text{CO}_2$ is characteristic, with a restrictive pattern of lung volumes. Withdrawal of the drug and steroid therapy can reverse the process.

*Busulphan* is an alkylating agent used in the treatment of chronic myeloid leukaemia. The drug can produce an insidious pulmonary infiltrate up to 10 years after starting treatment. Breathlessness may be associated with a low-grade fever and cough; the sputum often contains type II alveolar macrophages with atypical nuclei, which can be recognized by an expert cytologist. Opportunistic infection or radiation pneumonitis may be mimicked (see Chapter 8). A restrictive pattern of respiratory function with hypoxaemia results, the condition being progressive and irreversible once definite evidence of restriction has developed, but steroid therapy may halt the process if given in the earlier stages.

*Bleomycin*, an anti-tumour antibiotic used in treatment of Hogdkin's disease, leukaemia and some epidermoid carcinomas, can cause pulmonary fibrosis within six months of starting treatment. Older patients are more susceptible, and the pulmonary involvement appears to be dose-related. Cough and breathlessness are again characteristic, with infiltrates on the chest radiograph and development of a progressive irreversible restriction of lung volumes with hypoxaemia. A fall in TCO may be the earliest indication that toxicity is developing and high doses of steroids may then reverse the effects if the drug is withdrawn.

*Nitrofurantoin* is used in the treatment of urinary tract infections. The drug can cause both acute and chronic pulmonary toxicity. The *acute pulmonary reaction* consists of fever with chills and cyanosis associated with breathlessness, with a clinical picture resembling pulmonary oedema, developing within hours or days of starting the drug. Profuse basal infiltrates are seen on the radiograph and there is usually a blood eosinophilia. A *chronic pulmonary condition*, developing after treatment with nitrofurantoin for six months to six years can present as a low-grade fever with increasing breathlessness; again the radiograph shows bilateral basal fibrosis. However, in the chronic condition there is little blood eosinophilia. Pleural effusion may develop. Withdrawal of the drug and substitution of oral steroids may reverse the process.

# Pulmonary oedema

*Non-cardiogenic pulmonary oedema* (see Chapter 22) can arise from many causes. In that due to heroin abuse there may be clouding of consciousness, as well as the widespread crepitations of pulmonary oedema, along with the small pupils of the heroin addict and the marks of intravenous injections. This reaction of heroin-induced pulmonary oedema is a well recognized danger in the heroin addict who 'main-lines' the drug. Carbon dioxide retention is characteristic.

*Oxygen toxicity* can occur when breathing at atmospheric pressure if high concentrations of oxygen are breathed continuously for a prolonged time. The first symptoms are persistent cough with substernal pain, which is associated with a reduction in vital capacity, and this can arise even after 24 hours of continuously breathing oxygen in concentrations over 50%. At this early stage the condition can be rapidly reversed by a return to breathing air. However, if the oxygen breathing continues, progressive radiographic infiltrates herald the development of the adult respiratory distress syndrome (see Chapter 11). An increasing amount of the cardiac output is shunted through unventilated alveoli, so that the shunt fraction (see Chapter 3) increases, with the paradoxical development of increasing severity of arterial hypoxaemia, despite the administration of higher concentrations of oxygen in the inspired gas. This insoluble conundrum can be avoided by ensuring that oxygen concentrations higher than 40–50% are not breathed continuously. This risk presents only in patients being ventilated by a cuffed endotracheal tube.

*Paraquat*, a very powerful herbicide widely used in agriculture, is also a very powerful animal poison. The drug specifically damages the lungs by release of singlet oxygen ($O^-$), causing severe pulmonary oedema and haemorrhages, with a characteristic exuberant fibrosis with the formation of hyaline membranes. After a quiescent period marked by burning of the throat and lips after drinking paraquat, respiratory failure then ensues with diffuse infiltrates on the chest radiograph and hypoxaemia which rapidly becomes profound. This is usually associated with concomitant renal failure. Despite a plethora of effort, no therapy has yet been found consistently to reverse these devastating effects. It appears that the damage done by paraquat occurs during the first circulation of the poison after its rapid absorption. Lethal poisoning nearly always follows ingestion of the concentrated Gramoxone, which is sold only to farmers as a registered poison.

# Pulmonary hypertension

*Aminorex*, an appetite suppressant, had been linked epidemiologically with the remarkable outbreak of primary pulmonary hypertension in fat young women in German-speaking Europe. Although the disease cannot be reproduced in animals, the incidence fell dramatically when the drug was withdrawn from the market (see Chapter 18).

*Contraceptive pills* which contain a high dose of oestrogen (over 50 μg) have also been linked epidemiologically with an increased incidence of venous thrombosis and resultant pulmonary thrombo-embolism. This risk has led to a widespread change to low dosage oestrogen-progesterone pills, where the oestrogen dose is below 50 μg, and this appears to have minimized the risk. Nonetheless, any woman presenting with pulmonary thromboembolism should be asked if she is taking a contraceptive pill and, if so, advised to seek an alternative means of contraception.

# Drug-induced lupus syndromes

*Procainamide* is used in the treatment of ventricular tachycardia. The drug is well recognized to precipitate a lupus-like syndrome with pleuritic pain and pneumonic infiltrates, which are often associated with pleural effusion. The LE test is often positive and antinuclear factor is present in the serum. As well as the pulmonary lesions, arthropathy and low-grade fever are common. These side effects of procainamide may be slow to resolve after discontinuing the drug. *Hydrallazine* produces a similar reaction. As with many other pulmonary reactions to drugs, older patients appear to be more susceptible to side effects.

## Further reading

BREWIS, R. A. L. (1977) Respiratory disorders. In *Textbook of Adverse Drug Reactions*, ed. D. M. Davies. Oxford: Oxford University Press.

COLLIS, C. H. (1980) Lung damage from cytotoxic drugs. *Cancer Chemother. Pharmac.*, **4**, 17–27.

DUKES, M. N. G. (1980) *Meyler's Side Effects of Drugs*, 9th ed. Amsterdam: Excerpta Medica.

FRANK, L. and MASSARO, D. (1980) Oxygen toxicity. *Am. J. Med.*, **69**, 117–126.
PETRIE, J. C. (1980) *Clinically Important Adverse Drug Interactions, 1. Cardiovascular and Respiratory Disease Therapy.* Amsterdam: Elsevier/North Holland.
ROSENOW, E. C. (1972) Spectrum of drug-induced pulmonary disease. *Ann. intern. Med.*, **77**, 977–991.
SOSTMAN, H. D., MATTHAY, R. A. and PUTMAN, C. E. (1977) Cytotoxic drug-induced lung disease. *Am. J. Med.*, **62**, 608–615.
WEISS, R. A. and MUGGIA, F. M. (1980) Cytotoxic drug-induced pulmonary disease. *Am. J. Med.*, **68**, 259–265.

# 22

# Pulmonary Oedema

Pulmonary oedema means an increase in the volume of liquid lying outside the vascular bed of the lungs. This excess liquid can either occupy the interstitial space, lying between the vascular and alveolar compartments, forming interstitial oedema, or also flood the alveoli themselves, causing alveolar oedema.

## Cardiogenic pulmonary oedema

In practice, pulmonary oedema most often results from an increase in pulmonary venous hydrostatic pressure as a result of left heart failure, this being known as cardiogenic pulmonary oedema. This, in turn, can result from:

1. *Mitral valve disease*, as in mitral stenosis, with raised left atrial pressure, eventually leading to right ventricular hypertrophy; mitral incompetence, with left ventricular hypertrophy.

2. *Aortic valve disease* (either incompetence or stenosis), causing left ventricular hypertrophy, with displacement of the apex beat.

3. *Ischaemic heart disease*, particularly with myocardial infarction involving the left ventricle, where pulmonary oedema is a very common complication of acute myocardial infarction.

4. *Hypertensive heart* disease with left ventricular hypertrophy.

The clinical presentation of cardiogenic pulmonary oedema is well known, with breathlessness, often presenting as *paroxysmal nocturnal dyspnoea* (to be distinguished from that due to bronchial asthma), fine bilateral basal crepitations in the lung fields and pink frothy sputum. Clinical examination will go a long way towards establishing the cause of the cardiogenic pulmonary oedema, as indicated briefly above, and this may be confirmed by ECG and chest radiograph. The radiographic signs of pulmonary oedema include a selective dilatation of the upper lobe vessels, a perihilar haze, with Kerley B lines in the costophrenic angles (see Fig. 36), these all being characteristic of interstitial oedema. Frank alveolar pulmonary oedema can cause the well known 'bat's wing' distribution of alveolar infiltrates, based on the hilum on each side.

Whatever the underlying pathological cause of cardiogenic pulmonary oedema, treatment depends upon correction of the invariable hypoxaemia by high concentrations of oxygen, as the arterial $P\text{CO}_2$ is nearly always low in pulmonary oedema. Intravenous frusemide (40–80 mg) and parenteral morphine (10–15 mg, usually with 50 mg cyclizine) probably both act in part by reducing the central pulmonary blood volume, thus lowering the vascular pressures, an action which has been shown to occur before the characteristic diuresis develops. Morphine diminishes the respiratory drive, allowing the low arterial $P\text{CO}_2$ to return towards normal, any resulting tendency for aggravation of arterial hypoxaemia being corrected by the oxygen therapy. Left ventricular failure may merit therapy by intravenous digoxin, 0.25–0.5 mg, which is safe provided that no digoxin therapy has been given within the previous 14 days, followed by oral digoxin. Intravenous aminophylline also serves to lower vascular pressures by a vasodilator effect and potentiates the diuretic action of the frusemide.

# Non-cardiogenic pulmonary oedema

In health, fluid is driven out of the pulmonary capillaries into the interstitial space, through the capillary endothelium under the opposing forces of the capillary hydrostatic pressure and the colloid oncotic pressure of the plasma proteins, tending to draw the interstitial fluid back into the capillaries. Excess interstitial fluid is removed by lymphatics and it seems probable that the interstitial pressure within the lungs is, in fact, subatmospheric, although physiological debate continues as to the results of this difficult measurement in life. Nonetheless, these fundamental physiological principles must apply and depend upon the integrity of the pulmonary endothelium acting as a semipermeable membrane. If this endothelium is damaged, so allowing large molecular weight particles to pass across the endothelium, the colloid oncotic plasma protein pressure can no longer draw fluid back into the capillaries from the interstitial space and pulmonary oedema will develop. Obviously, a fall in concentration of the plasma proteins themselves, particularly the albumin fraction, will also contribute to reduction of such colloid oncotic pressure, leading potentially to pulmonary oedema. Thus, in practice, non-cardiogenic pulmonary oedema can result from:

1. Viral, bacterial or aspiration pneumonia damaging the pulmonary endothelium.

2. Inhaled toxic agents, e.g. phosgene, nitrous fumes, smoke, near-drowning.

3. Circulating toxic agents, as in bacteraemic shock, paraquat lung, histamine, snake venoms, etc.

4. Disseminated intravascular coagulation.

5. Uraemia.
6. Radiation pneumonitis.
7. Post-traumatic pulmonary insufficiency or shock lung.

The pulmonary oedema in these situations manifests as the adult respiratory distress syndrome (see Chapter 11).

In *hypoalbuminaemia*, as in the nephrotic syndrome, cirrhosis of the liver, protein–energy malnutrition, protein-losing enteropathy, etc., chronic pulmonary oedema is always a potential complication. Hypoxaemia in these conditions, with a widening of the alveolar to arterial oxygen tension gradient (A-a$DO_2$), particularly when the patient is sitting upright, probably results from closure of small airways at the bases of the lungs, so that alveoli in these regions are no longer ventilated, yet still perfused. This airway closure results from oedema fluid forming a perivascular cuff within the pulmonary lobules, around the respiratory bronchioles and their accompanying arterioles, so causing airway closure. This is probably of little clinical consequence unless the hypoalbuminaemia becomes profound, but it must be recognized that further fluid overload in such patients can lead to more overt pulmonary oedema, particularly if there is a degree of left ventricular failure from associated myocardial ischaemia for example.

*High-altitude pulmonary oedema*, a life-threatening condition, has been increasingly recognized in recent years, from its first widespread description in the war between India and China, when armies faced each other, possibly for the first time in history, at over 4000 m above sea level. The clinical picture is now also well recognized in mountaineers and skiers and consists of acute pulmonary oedema, with prodromata of oliguria, headache, giddiness and insomnia, which occurs in previously fit subjects who have ascended rapidly to over 4000 m in altitude and have carried out relatively severe muscular exercise shortly after arrival at altitude. Mountaineers and skiers who have arrived at altitude by air are clearly potential victims. The pulmonary oedema usually develops around the third day at altitude, but responds rapidly to oxygen and frusemide, and can be prevented adequately by taking prophylactic acetazolamide, 250 mg daily by mouth.

Pulmonary oedema can also result from *heroin over-dosage* (see Chapter 19).

*Neurogenic pulmonary oedema* is a rare but recognized complication of an acutely raised intracranial pressure, as in head injury, subarachnoid haemorrhage, cerebral tumour, etc. It is possible that the pulmonary oedema results from a rise in pulmonary vascular pressures from stimulation of sympathetic vasomotor centres in the medulla.

Treatment of non-cardiogenic pulmonary oedema is essentially symptomatic, depending upon oxygen, diuretics and morphine. Advanced cases with endothelial capillary damage presenting as the adult respiratory distress syndrome are managed as described in Chapter 11.

## Further reading

SNASHALL, P. D. (1980) Pulmonary oedema. *Br. J. Dis. Chest*, **74**, 2–22.

# 23

# Mediastinal Masses

The mediastinum, like Julius Caesar's Gaul, is divided into three parts (Fig. 85). Mediastinal masses can occur at any age, but are characteristically associated with three different mediastinal positions, so that a lateral chest radiograph is often the most important initial diagnostic measure.

## Anterior compartment

Masses in the anterior compartment are most likely to be due to *thymoma* (20% of all mediastinal masses), which may present with cough, chest pain or superior vena caval obstruction. Myasthenia gravis occurs in 10–50% of patients with a thymoma. Red blood cell aplasia and hypogammaglobulinaemia are other recognized but rare associations. Thymomata are clearly outlined dense opacities occurring near the junction of the heart and great vessels, calcification being seen in some 20%. Surgical excision is recommended, as the tumour may be malignant.

*Dermoid cysts* (benign teratomata) are usually symptomless unless infection or malignant change develops. Men are at most risk of malignant change in this tumour, which can account of some 15% of mediastinal masses. Dermoids appear as dense, homogeneous lobular shadows in the anterior mediastinum, often with calcification in the walls, and teeth may be recognized within the tumour. Surgical removal is always recommended, in view of the potential of malignant change. *Primary teratomata* are malignant tumours, at the same site as the dermoid tumour, the lesions being always solid. Radiation therapy following surgery is recommended.

*Hodgkin's disease* or non-Hodgkin's lymphomas can present rarely as mediastinal masses, from involvement of mediastinal lymph nodes.

*Intrathoracic goitres* are anterior mediastinal lesions which may occur particularly in middle-aged women, who are usually asymptomatic. Stridor, hoarseness and dysphagia, however, are all recognized presenting features. The true nature of the lesion is sometimes revealed by a radio-active iodine scan. Treatment is surgical.

239

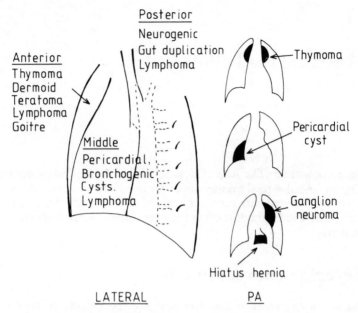

*Fig. 85.*   Common positions of mediastinal masses of different origin, as seen on the lateral radiograph and possible presentations on the posteroanterior chest radiograph

# Middle mediastinum

The middle mediastinum is the site of *pleuropericardial cysts* ('spring water cysts'), characteristically appearing as a smooth sharply-demarcated mass of uniform density at the right cardiophrenic angle. Surgical excision may be necessary if other potentially malignant tumours at this site cannot be excluded by previous chest film, or ultra-sound. Bronchogenic cysts and reduplication of the oesophagus are other rare causes of masses in the middle mediastinum.

# Posterior mediastinum

*Neurogenic tumours*, although rare, are the commonest of all mediastinal tumours and characteristically arise in the posterior mediastinum, along the paravertebral gutter. These tumours are often asymptomatic in the adult, but may cause chest pain, with stridor, breathlessness, cough and tracheal compression. Horner's syndrome or spinal cord compression can occur. The characteristic radiographical appearance shows a well circumscribed round mass in the posterior mediastinum, possibly with widening of the adjacent rib spaces. As with other mediastinal masses, surgical excision is recommended, often followed by radiotherapy if the resected specimen shows clear evidence of malignant change. *Generalized neurofibromatosis* occurs in about one-quarter of patients with a primary posterior mediastinal neurofibroma. Catecholamine secretion can be associated with the rare phaeochromocytomata in the posterior mediastinum, or with other neurogenic tumours.

## Further reading

WYCHULIS, A. R., PAYNE, W. S., CLAGETT, O. T. and WOOLNER, L. B. (1971) Surgical treatment of mediastinal tumours. *J. thorac. cardiovasc. Surg.*, **62**, 379–392.

# 24

# Miscellaneous Topics

## Sleep apnoea

Cessation of breathing during sleep has attracted great attention recently, it now being recognized as temporary apnoea with breathing suspended for 10 seconds or more, and is by no means uncommon from time to time during a normal healthy night's sleep. These episodes become more frequent in older subjects, and occur most frequently during the rapid eye movement (REM) phase of sleep, when dreaming occurs. When such episodes occur more frequently than four to five times for each hour of sleep, the patient is said to be suffering from a *sleep apnoea syndrome*. These are divided into *obstructive apnoea*, when chest wall and diaphragmatic movement appear to continue, although there is no air flow occurring at the nose and mouth, indicating that the upper airway is temporary occluded; and *central apnoea*, where the problem appears to arise from transient failure of central respiratory drive.

### Obstructive sleep apnoea

Although apparently rare, this syndrome is being increasingly recognized and is characterized by snoring and abnormal movements during sleep, with day-time headache and sleepiness. Progressive failure of intellectual function can occur, often leading to serious social consequences. The disease has been recognized in children and may be related to the *sudden infant death syndrome* ('cot death') in which children aged between three months and one year are found unexpectedly dead in their cots. Obstructive sleep apnoea in the adult appears principally to be a disease of men and post-menopausal women. Patients are often obese, with a short thick neck, and the syndrome has clearly been documented to occur in a variety of neurological and congenital abnormalities of the upper airway including malocclusion of the teeth. During the apnoeic episodes, which may occur up to two or more times per hour of sleep, loud snoring occurs, indicating partial upper airway obstruction. The snoring suddenly ceases and progressive hypoxaemia then rapidly develops, with a

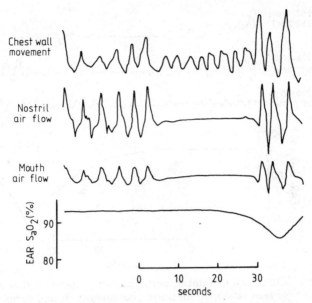

Chest wall
movement

Nostril
air flow

Mouth
air flow

EAR S$_a$O$_2$ (%)

90

80

0    10    20    30
seconds

*Fig. 86.*    Chest wall movement, nostril air flow, mouth air flow and ear
oxygen saturation measured continuously during a period of
obstructive sleep apnoea

marked tendency to cardiac arrhythmias and a definite incidence of
sudden death. The condition may masquerade as narcolepsy and
patients have often been to a series of specialists, including neurol-
ogists and psychiatrists, before the real nature of their disorder has
been recognized. The diagnosis is established by recording the chest
wall movements, air flow at nose and mouth, ear oxygen saturation,
ECG and EEG continuously throughout one or two nights of sleep
(Fig. 86). These studies are carried out in a special sleep laboratory.
Systemic and pulmonary hypertension can complicate the condition
and this can progress to obstructive cor pulmonale. This latter has long
been recognized as a rare consequence of marked *hypertrophy of the
adenoids and tonsils* in children, but it is now known that such
hypertrophy can present with upper airway obstruction and sleep
apnoea. The physiological mechanisms underlying the airway obstruction seem to depend upon failure of the normal reflex activation of
the muscle dilators of the pharynx. During normal sleep these muscles
contract during inspiration and so keep the upper airway open. This
mechanism appears to fail in obstructive sleep apnoea, so that the
upper airway becomes occluded.

*Treatment* depends upon relieving the airway obstruction.

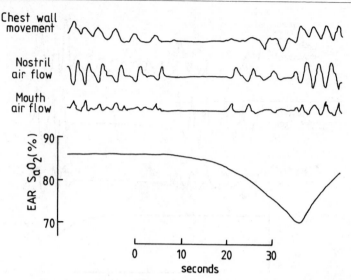

*Fig. 87.*    Chest wall movement, nostril air flow, mouth air flow and ear oxygen saturation measured continuously during an episode of central sleep apnoea. Note cessation of air flow for more than 10 sections, both nose and mouth, with absence of chest wall movement

Although this can be achieved by loss of weight, and possibly by medroxyprogesterone acetate (100–200 mg daily) or protriptyline, permanent tracheostomy has been proved to be an effective and acceptable treatment in patients with severe intellectual disorders as a result of obstructive sleep apnoea. However, the published number of such patients is still small and the author of these studies has emphasized that careful selection of patients and expert psychological and social support are essential if success is to be obtained from this procedure.

## Central sleep apnoea

This is less common than obstructive apnoea and much less well understood physiologically. The condition is probably related to the *sudden infant death syndrome* (SIDS) and adult members of families in which SIDS has occurred have been described as suffering occasionally from central sleep apnoea. Children who survived a 'near-miss' episode were found on monitoring of their sleep to have recurrence of central apnoea and it seems probable that the central mechanisms controlling the regulation of respiration during sleep, particularly during the REM (Fig. 87), are not usually fully developed at birth. These mechanisms appear to develop physiologically over the next six months to one year, for if a child who has had a 'near-miss' from SIDS can be kept alive for this period by use of an apnoea alarm to indicate to the parents the necessity for resuscitation, it seems that the condition itself is overcome as the child grows older.

# Mycetoma

A mycetoma (aspergilloma) is the name given to a large colony of *Aspergillus fumigatus* which grows within a pre-existing cavity within the lungs. This usually results from an old tuberculous cavity, but can also occur in a bronchiectatic cavity and rarely in a cavitated neoplasm or pulmonary infarct. Haemoptysis, which can be severe and life-threatening, is usually the only symptom. A mycetoma is often detected only on the chest radiograph, where it appears as a solid opacity within a previously known cavity, with the characteristic crescent of air separating the fungus ball from the wall of the cavity. This is best shown by tomography of the lesion (Fig. 88). The wall of the cavity is usually adherent to the fungus ball at some point. The wall contains vascular granulomatous tissue, thus accounting for the marked tendency to haemoptysis. Skin tests (indicating circulating specific IgE) are positive in less than half of these cases, but IgG, shown as precipitins within the serum to *Aspergillus*, is present in 80% of cases. Treatment is difficult as curative lobectomy is usually prevented both by the extent of lung involved (bilateral mycetoma being known) and by the patient's poor respiratory function. The sputum nearly always contains fungal mycelial elements and culture of the *Aspergillus* from sputum often yields several variant strains. This is shown by their colony characteristics and can be an indicator that mycelial elements in the sputum are indeed derived from a mycetoma. The differential diagnosis lies between reactivation of tuberculosis, or the apparently solid lesion on the radiograph may at first be thought to be a bronchial carcinoma, particularly if the patient presents with haemoptysis.

# Pulmonary eosinophilia

Eosinophil granulocytes are closely involved in both Type I (IgE-initiated immune reactions), where they are attracted by the ECF-A release by degranulating mast cells, and also in immune complex reactions (Type III). Peripheral blood eosinophilia is characteristic clinically of atopic asthma, enteric worm infestation and many skin disorders and is commonly associated with high levels of circulating IgE. The association of radiographically evident lung infiltrates with

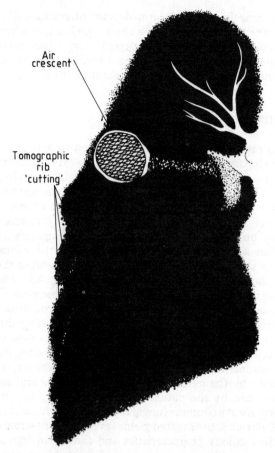

*Fig. 88.*     Sketch of a posteroanterior tomogram of the chest showing the air crescent surrounding an apsergilloma lying in a lung cavity

an excess of eosinophils in both sputum and peripheral blood is known as pulmonary eosinophilia.

*Simple pulmonary eosinophilia (Loeffler's syndrome)* is a short-lived illness usually associated with intestinal worms (*Ascaris lumbricoides, Ankylostoma, Trichuris, Taenia saginata*) or numerous drugs including aspirin, penicillin, sulphonamides, etc. There may be no symptoms, the condition being discovered on routine chest radiography, or the patient may complain of cough, mild fever and muscular aches, wheezing and dyspnoea being uncommon. Peripheral transient opacities in the chest radiograph are characteristic, the condition usually clearing completely within two to four weeks.

*Prolonged pulmonary eosinophilia* is less common, sometimes seen particularly in middle-aged housewives. These patients may be more ill than those with simple Loeffler's syndrome, with cough and mucoid sputum and some breathlessness and occasionally high fever. Tuberculosis may be mimicked. Axillary or apical radiographic infiltrates are often seen in these patients and these are usually based on the pleura and not upon the hilum. In addition to eosinophilia (which is not always present in the peripheral blood, but is always seen in the sputum), the ESR is raised and hypoxaemia with a widening of $A–aDO_2$ may be present.

Blood abnormalities and radiographic changes usually resolve rapidly after prednisolone 20 mg daily has been started, but a maintenance dose of steroids may be necessary to prevent recurrence.

*Asthmatic pulmonary eosinophilia* is the commonest variety of these disorders and is nearly always due to *allergic bronchopulmonary aspergillosis*. Transient radiographic infiltrates may be due to collapse of lung behind a plug of inspirated mucus, which is often packed with mycelial elements of *Aspergillus*. Proximal bronchiectasis is characteristic, but the *Aspergillus* rarely invades the bronchial wall. Tubular and ring shadows may persist when the dense opacities resolve, indicating permanent thickening of bronchial walls. Diagnosis can be confirmed by immediate skin reactions to *Aspergillus* (Type I reactions) and by the finding of aspergillin precipitins (IgA immune complex) in the serum. Treatment depends upon oral steroids, with prednisolone in a dose of at least 20 mg daily or maybe higher to control the asthmatic reaction, progress being monitored by a clearing of radiographic infiltrates and by improvement in $FEV_1$, which is nearly always impaired in these patients initially.

*Tropical pulmonary eosinophilia* results from filarial infestation, being encountered in India, south-east Asia, tropical Africa and South America. Cough, wheeze, dyspnoea and chest pain are characteristic and fever and weight loss may also occur, the radiograph characteristically showing mottling in both lung fields in middle and lower zones. The IgE concentration in the serum is very high and eosinophil counts are usually over $3000/mm^3$. Diethylcarbamazine 6 mg/kg daily in three divided doses given for three weeks, starting with a dose of 1 mg/kg and increasing to the 6 mg/kg dose over three days, is effective. Pulmonary fibrosis can develop if the condition is not treated.

Eosinophilia with pulmonary infiltrates can also occur in *drug reactions* (see Chapter 21) and in *collagen vascular diseases* (see Chapter 19).

## Further reading

GUILLEMINAULT, C. and DEMENT, W. C. (1978) *Sleep Apnea Syndromes.* New York: Alan R. List

LIEBOW, A. A. and CARRINGTON, C. B. (1968) The eosinophilic pneumonias. *Medicine, Balt.,* **48**, 251–285.

PENNINGTON, J. E. (1980) *Aspergillus* lung disease. In symposium on infectious lung diseases. *Med. Clins N. Am.,* **64**, 475–490.

# Index